FOSTERING MENTAL HEALTH LITERACY THROUGH ADOLESCENT LITERATURE

FOSTERING MENTAL HEALTH LITERACY THROUGH ADOLESCENT LITERATURE

Edited by
Brooke Eisenbach
Jason Scott Frydman

ROWMAN & LITTLEFIELD
Lanham • Boulder • New York • London

Published by Rowman & Littlefield
An imprint of The Rowman & Littlefield Publishing Group, Inc.
4501 Forbes Boulevard, Suite 200, Lanham, Maryland 20706
www.rowman.com

6 Tinworth Street, London, SE11 5AL, United Kingdom

British Library Cataloguing in Publication Information Available

Library of Congress Cataloging-in-Publication Data

Names: Eisenbach, Brooke, editor. | Frydman, Jason Scott, 1983– editor.
Title: Fostering mental health literacy through adolescent literature /
    edited by Brooke Eisenbach, Jason Scott Frydman.
Description: Lanham, Maryland : Rowman & Littlefield, [2021] | Includes
    index. | Summary: "This collection provides secondary (6–12) educators
    with background information pertaining to a variety of mental health themes,
    along with specific pedagogical approaches for engaging readers in
    developing their mental health literacy"—Provided by publisher.
Identifiers: LCCN 2021030036 (print) | LCCN 2021030037 (ebook) | ISBN
    9781475858792 (Cloth : acid-free paper) | ISBN 9781475858808 (Paperback
    : acid-free paper) | ISBN 9781475858815 (ePub)
Subjects: LCSH: Content area reading—Study and teaching
    (Secondary)—United States. | Mental health education—United States.
Classification: LCC LB1050.455 .F68 2021 (print) | LCC LB1050.455 (ebook)
    | DDC 362.2071—dc23
LC record available at https://lccn.loc.gov/2021030036
LC ebook record available at https://lccn.loc.gov/2021030037

Brooke dedicates this book to Olivia.
You inspire me each and every day.
I love you for all that you are and all that you will ever be.
I am so proud to be your mommy.

Jason dedicates this book to JP and Laura.
You make the world go round and the many moments still.
You each supply my motivation and consideration.
Love you always.

CONTENTS

INTRODUCTION

Preparing to Engage with Mental Health Themes in Adolescent Literature

Jason Scott Frydman and Brooke Eisenbach

Adolescence is a time of notable transitions. Biopsychosocial shifts occur that bring about a heightened sense of self and social awareness, leading to an exploration of peer relationships, identity formation, and autonomy. During this time, active engagement with the world intersects with a susceptibility to social and biological influences that have the potential to manifest as mental health struggles or diagnosable psychiatric disorders (Zhao et al., 2015). In understanding the exact prevalence of this occurrence, data show that one in six youth in the United States has some form of serious emotional, behavioral, or other mental health need (National Alliance on Mental Illness [NAMI], 2021). Furthermore, half of all lifetime cases of mental illnesses begin by age 14, with the majority emerging prior to adulthood (Merikangas et al., 2010; NAMI, 2021). As adolescents struggle with mental health challenges, and associated stigmas, they are at an increased risk for negative socio-emotional and academic outcomes, all while undergoing concurrent developmental transitions (Deighton et al., 2018; McLeod, Uemura, & Rohrman, 2012; Moses, 2010). Due to these inherent changes in adolescence and their resultant vulnerabilities, there is a need to promote knowledge of mental health to generate awareness, reduce stigma, and normalize individual and peer experiences.

School districts throughout the country are beginning to seek out ways of introducing and navigating mental health education within middle and high school classrooms. Notably, a growing trend has been to legally mandate a mental health curriculum state-wide. For example, in 2018, New York and Virginia became the first two states to pass a law that requires mental health instruction for comprehensive programming in schools (Vestal, 2018), focusing on K–12 (New York) and a more targeted adolescent cohort of 9th and 10th graders (Virginia). Florida was the third state to follow suite, passing a 2019 bill that enforces an instructional focus on mental health needs for 6th through 12th graders (Florida Department of Education, 2019). This movement is beginning to rapidly expand across the country. In 2019, Nevada appropriated funding for mental health education to be provided by school-based professionals (Nevada SB204, 2019), Texas passed a law that will require teachers to receive instruction in mental health education to satisfy professional certification requirements (Texas HB18, 2019), and Colorado released sizable funding to train teachers in suicide prevention and crisis management (Colorado SB18-272, 2019).

As educators search for ways to effectively enrich the social and emotional development of adolescent learners and eliminate stigma surrounding mental illness, adolescent literature can serve as a starting point for connection, reflection, and education. To support students in this way, teachers need to first provide meaningful instruction that raises awareness of these topics. This book is a collection of chapters seeking to promote adolescent learning through *mental health literacy*, or the "knowledge and beliefs about mental disorders which aid their recognition, management, or prevention" (Jorm, 2000). Recent scholarship has touted the immense opportunity that fiction holds in educating adolescents on mental health issues (Aziz et al., 2019; Hall, 2020; Moore & Begoray, 2017; Richmond, 2014, 2019). This developing consensus within the education field posits that the use of adolescent literature in the English language arts (ELA) classroom promotes both recognition and understanding, key elements in counteracting the negative impact of public and peer stigma surrounding mental health (Corrigan et al., 2012; O'Driscoll et al., 2012). In fact, research suggests that educational programming aimed at reducing mental health stigma has proven particularly effective with adolescents (Corrigan et al., 2012); adolescents have demonstrably shown that exposure to information leads to behavioral change (Montgomery & Maunders, 2015; Milin et al., 2016). This finding, that education can support both measurable learning outcomes and motivate action, is the driving factor underlying this text.

At its core, literature can serve as a starting point for conversation and activity that centers the academic while enhancing the social and emotional growth of learners. Reading mental health–based adolescent literature in the middle or high school classroom, along with activities designed to enhance readers' mental health education, can increase empathy and mental health awareness. The chapters in this book provide insight on the prevalence and performance of mental health issues among an adolescent population. In the initial eight chapters, this includes in-depth descriptions and educational activities that consider a variety of mental health issues, including: adverse experiences of rural life, loss and grief, eating disorders, trauma exposure and the transgenerational transmission of trauma, substance and opioid use, depression and suicide, and obsessive-compulsive disorder. The final chapter, which highlights the use of book clubs to promote mental health literacy, presents a series of books that offer additional mental health foci, for example, self-harm, sexual abuse, anxiety, schizoaffective disorder, hallucinations, hoarding, bipolar disorder, anger issues, and schizophrenia. Author teams, which are intentionally composed of educators and mental health professionals, highlight how fictional characters experience mental health issues personally and in relationship to others.

Within this text, mental health is explored from both a macro and micro perspective. On a macro-level, chapters provide descriptive statistics that shape a broader understanding of each featured mental health topic as it applies to adolescents. Balancing this overview are the micro-level experiences of fictional adolescent characters who are navigating their unique mental health struggles; therefore, this text sits at the crossroads of real-world adolescent mental health and the heightened reality of literary fiction; the combination of which provides an access point for students to explore more fully a comprehensive and nuanced understanding of mental health, enhancing their literacy on the topic.

THE STRUCTURE OF THIS TEXT

The structure of each chapter is uniform for ease of reference and accessibility. Chapters are broken down into six sections: introduction, summary of the book, before-reading strategies, during-reading strategies, after-reading strategies, and conclusion. The introduction section orients teachers to the mental health topic with foundational knowledge and relevant statistics that can be used as source material, while also introducing an ELA focus for the individual text.

Following a brief summary of the book, the before-reading strategies (titled "Guiding Students into the Text" in each chapter) outlines key definitions of relevant mental health terms and instructional strategies to prepare students for both the mental health topic and literacy focus. These strategies are intended to support learners for encountering mental health issues by providing preemptive information and introduce a specific literacy skill that will then carry over into the during-reading activities (titled "Guiding Students through the Text" in each chapter).

As students journey through the text, chapters provide teachers pedagogical activities to enhance readers' mental health literacy while further developing specific reading literacy skills such as character analysis, examination of theme, and plot development. During-reading strategies are designed to deepen the understanding of the mental health topic as represented through the lens, or lenses, of the fictional character(s) they encounter. Specific lessons are designed to teach the featured literacy skill or concept through applied exercises to strengthen textual analysis and student reading engagement. Additionally, to reconcile textual content, this section features a series of discussion questions meant to activate critical thinking and integration of both ELA and mental health themes.

To reinforce their disciplinary literacy development and demonstrate accrued mental health literacy, after-reading strategies (titled "Guiding Students out of the Text" in each chapter) are provided to transform education into application. At their close, chapters offer a "Call to Action," section wherein teachers are given ideas to support students proactively transitioning their acquired mental health literacy beyond the classroom walls. Through scaffolded activities that build from the before- and during-reading sections, students are guided in a collaborative process on ways to educate others on what they have learned, solidifying their own understanding and becoming agents of change.

SUGGESTIONS FOR GETTING STARTED

Cultivating a "Person-Centered" Classroom Community

Teaching is a profession that carries both instructional and relational responsibilities. Research has revealed that caring relationships are foundational to a strong educational environment (Lake et al., 2014; Owusu-Ansah & Kyei-Blankson, 2016). Before engaging students in reading, discussion, and activity surrounding matters of mental health and/or mental illness, it is imperative to establish a classroom community of inclusivity and choice. For the purpose of enhancing students' mental health literacy and normalizing mental health issues/illness, teachers should first give attention to a "person-centered" approach to community building. Such an approach centers classroom conditions for empathy, genuineness, and positive regard for the social-emotional growth of all learners (Rogers, 1961; Range et al., 2013).

As a means of facilitating a person-centered classroom community, we encourage the adoption of a "brave spaces" framework (Arao & Clemens, 2013). Establishing a safe space in a classroom is often intended to ensure that students do not feel marginalized or excluded based on their personal identifiers in relation to a topic or discussion; however, classroom content may feature concepts or activities that may make students unintentionally, or at times intentionally, feel challenged, potentially undermining the initial purpose of the safe space. In response, the brave space context is an extension of a safe space with the added goal of welcoming differences and clarifying conversations, centering on the following five elements for dialogue: maintaining civility while allowing for unique perspectives, acknowledging individual and subjective responses, providing the option to move in and out of participation around specific topics, maintaining an ongoing disposition of respect, and avoiding intentional interpersonal harm (Ali, 2017). In seeking to establish a brave space within a person-centered approach to community and instruction, teachers can focus on the building and sustaining of relationships and connections within the classroom, enhancing student voice, individual responses, and critical interpretation of text, all while promoting meaningful engagement with texts and activities (Range et al., 2013).

The stories shared through each book and activity center on characters experiencing mental health needs or mental illness. As such, it is important that students feel connected and respected before engaging in this critical work. As students partake in activities that require the unpacking of potential bias, stigma, and misinformation, it is important they feel the classroom community is a brave space that promotes inclusivity in speaking up and speaking out on these important matters.

Connecting with a Mental Health Professional

As teachers prepare to introduce texts and engage learners in matters of mental health literacy, we echo previous literature and strongly recommend connecting and collaborating with a school-based mental health professional (Moore & Begoray, 2017). This might mean teachers connect with the school's counselor, social worker, or psychologist to review the ideas and activities featured in a selected chapter, sharing one's intentions and plans for the reading and discussion of select course texts and/or materials, and finding ways to collaborate on instructional plans, preparation, and classroom activity. Teachers and mental health specialists can work together to identify additional resources for classroom use, as well as outside mental health resources. We also recommend inviting the mental health professional into the classroom to initiate the unit of study, at select intervals throughout the study of the text, and at the conclusion of the unit of study. If necessary, teachers can set a plan for referral for students who demonstrate a specific need for mental health support as the class engages in this work together.

Maintaining the Role of Classroom Teacher

Teachers may have a limited scope of knowledge of mental health and/or mental illness. As such, it is imperative to maintain one's role as classroom teacher, rather than take on the persona of counselor or therapist while navigating students through the texts and activities contained in this volume. Each chapter is purposefully the collaborative work of educators specialized in literacy and a mental health professional; however, the focus of this text is not on supporting therapeutic conversations or interventions in the classroom setting by classroom teachers. In line with a public health approach in schools to provide psychoeducation, this text is intended to promote literacy of mental health issues and illnesses through information sharing and representation within the books featured in each chapter. As such, the chapters are designed to provide teachers background information and insight into each of the noted mental health needs, while maintaining a clear focus on utilizing the suggested titles to introduce, teach, and reinforce particular skills and concepts within the ELA curriculum. Teachers should focus on questions and exploration of themes that speak directly to the text, rather than promote questions or activities that seek a personal mental health–related response.

It is important to note that some of the content in a book featured in this text may generate individual sharing by students. Establishing connections to literature can be critical in promoting comprehension, learning, and engagement for adolescent readers (Rosenblatt, 2005); however, openly discussing personal mental health issues in a classroom setting requires setting a clear framework for doing so, ensuring a brave space, and obtaining consent for such a conversation from the students (Ali, 2017; Moore & Begoray, 2017; Substance Abuse and Mental Health Services Administration [SAMHSA], 2014). Moreover, developmentally, adolescents are actively coordinating their cognition and affect (Casey & Caudle, 2013); this potential imbalance may yield unexpected emotional responses for which the boundaries of the classroom may be inappropriate. At the same time, while we encourage teachers to continually frame dialogue so that it is grounded in the content of the book, shutting down conversations centered on personal experiences can counteract the advocacy of this text. We therefore offer that the intentional or organic onset of such conversation would best be moderated with the presence and support of the school's mental health professional. As previously noted, one way to potentially prepare for these conversations is to evaluate the lessons in this text alongside the mental health support person and plan for classroom visits at strategic times or coordinate availability when engaged in teaching from the selected text.

Teachers should be mindful of potentially broaching the divide between the roles of teacher and mental health counselor. Should students seek mental health support, we suggest teachers reach out to the school mental health professional for available resources as a means of supporting students. *Teachers should not attempt to provide therapy or explicit mental health support within the classroom or with students.* Such interventions should be handled by mental health professionals who are specially trained and authorized to provide this type of support. Moreover, therapeutic engagement relies on maintaining boundaries and establishing a sense of mutual trust and sharing predicated on the therapist's assumed objectivity. While teachers can and often do function in a mentorship role for students, invoking a therapeutic frame can blur boundaries and potentially cause unintentional harm; therefore, we strongly suggest using the chapters to stimulate and enhance students' mental health literacy, rather than allowing the ideas to serve as a form of therapy or mental health support.

CONSIDERATIONS IN TEXT SELECTION

The adolescent texts shared throughout this volume were selected for middle or high school learners within the ELA classroom. As teachers seek out independent titles for the classroom, we offer the following suggestions to consider in the selection and evaluation of classroom text and material.

Consider Your Unique Classroom and Context

Every educator who engages in this work does so within a unique classroom community and context. As teachers cultivate a classroom of care, we encourage using knowledge of the students, their families, and the school community to select texts that are fitting for the needs, interests, cultures, identities, and abilities of the students in the classroom.

Avoid the Single Narrative in Sharing Stories and Experiences

It is crucial for students to understand that a single story cannot speak to a universal experience. The experiences and identity of one character are strictly that—the experiences and identity of that single character. Embrace a variety of texts that promote diverse perspectives, identities, and experiences.

Identify Diverse, Multidimensional Characters

Characters should not be defined by their mental illness. In one's search for additional titles, be critical of works that appear to define or depict characters through a narrow or singular lens. Ensure characters are multidimensional.

Critically Examine the Text and Research and Learn More about the Author(s)

Get to know more about the author of the text. Today, many authors are speaking up about their personal struggles with mental health in an effort to further normalize mental illness. While no author should be expected to share their story with the world, it can be informative and further the goals of this work to take the time to learn more about the experience of the writer and inspiration for the book.

In addition, it is important to examine each text with a critical lens. How is the author approaching mental health issues throughout the text? How are they representing mental health issues/illness within the text? Are they honest in the reflection of a need for ongoing treatment or management, or do they speak of a "magical cure"? Is the representation of mental illness portrayed as one with a positive or healthy course, rather than imminent tragedy? Teachers should ensure the texts selected for the classroom promote a positive exploration of mental health and treatment, rather than those that further bias, stereotypes, or stigmatization.

Consider Potential Triggers for Students and Yourself

Finally, teachers should be aware of potential triggers for students, and for oneself, in the selection of class texts. While the teacher will not be fully aware of every trigger for every student, as it is not the student's responsibility to share their private experience and identity, if teachers are aware that content or aspects of the story might prove potentially harmful or unsettling for readers, they should prepare for ways to navigate this moment in the classroom. At the same time, teachers should be honest in reflecting upon their personal experience and how the story might in some way trigger their own emotional response.

THE COLLECTION: CHAPTER FOCUS AND ORGANIZATION

The following chapter descriptions are contributions adapted from each author team to provide teachers with an overview of the mental health issue(s) and ELA standards featured throughout this text.

Our text opens with Jeff Spanke and Sara Tyner's focus on multimodal approaches to literacy instruction and examination of symbolism as featured in Kristin Russell's *A Sky for Us Alone* (2019). This adolescent novel resists the cultural narrative that mental health issues are unique to particular regions of particular people, and that certain "other" regions are somehow exempt from the perils (and treatment) of things like trauma, grief, and addiction. In this chapter, Spanke and Tyner examine how Russell's teen characters, as a means of coping with the grief, addiction, and loss of their respective circumstances, have themselves become parentified, as well as how the adults in their community reflect the needs of millions of Americans who may not know there's life outside the mines.

At some point, everyone, including young people, will experience the death of a loved one. Bereaved adolescents often look to their friends for support as they grieve. Sherri Harper Woods and Terry Benton's chapter uses Jason Reynolds's *The Boy in the Black Suit* (2015) to enhance students' mental health literacy concerning loss and the grieving process. Through an examination of characterization in the novel, adolescents can learn about types of loss, and subsequent grief, and the ways the characters experience loss within the story. Teachers can use the instructional strategies shared in this chapter to help students develop their understanding of character development in tandem with enhancing their ability to recognize the nuances of loss, symptoms of grief, and strategies in navigating the grieving process.

Eating disorders, disordered eating, and body image issues often begin during middle school and affect youth of all genders. As we live in a health-obsessed culture that celebrates body perfection, further exacerbated by social media, the need for preventative mental health literacy around food and body image issues with this age group is crucial. Laura L. Wood, MaryBeth DeGennaro, and Brooke Eisenbach use the text *Good Enough*, by Jen Petro-Roy (2019), and the Health at Every Size principles, to support teachers in having brave conversations with students about the worth of every person's body, while using the text to look at literacy devices such as point of view, characterization, metaphor, and simile.

Daniela Bustamante and Katie Sciurba address concepts of primary trauma, transgenerational trauma, and grief in their examination of Erika L. Sánchez's (2017) novel *I Am Not Your Perfect Mexican Daughter*. This chapter highlights silence and secrecy as trauma responses affecting characters throughout the novel. Given the context of multiple traumas and losses affecting the characters, as well as the ways in which Mexican (and Mexican American) culture shapes their complex identities, Bustamante and Sciurba's chapter offers teachers an avenue for exploring character development and conflict. The authors provide a variety of teaching activities, including jigsaws, debates, and writing exercises, to prepare students for content they will encounter in the book and to serve as guides for students to analyze the text. This chapter will help students develop a vocabulary for discussing and understanding concepts related to trauma and loss, identify sources and indicators of internal and external conflict, and map character development as they engage with the literature.

Hey, Kiddo, the National Book Award finalist graphic memoir by Jarrett Krosoczka (2018), chronicles the impact of addiction on a family. For this chapter, Grace Enriquez and Michelle Pate guide teachers and students through Krosoczka's graphic memoir as he uses art to heal and process his mother's struggles with substance use disorder. Specifically, the authors highlight the unique qualities of plot in memoir and visual storytelling in graphic format. With this lens, the authors provide space for teachers and students to explore how the trajectories of plot and graphic storytelling provide an honest depiction of the complexities of a family impacted by substance use disorder.

Elsie Lindy Olan, Kia Jane Richmond, and Mary Mae Kelly guide teachers and students into meaningful discussion and safe exploration of depression and suicidal ideation as shared in Cindy L. Rodriguez's (2015) *When Reason Breaks*. In this chapter, the authors provide teachers a series of activities designed to help students navigate biases and preconceived notions while analyzing characters' emotions and behaviors in the novel. Olan, Richmond, and Kelly provide activities designed to support students' acquisition of new knowledge via research and presentations, intentional reading practices, and activities to facilitate their responses to the text as they develop a better sense of mental health literacy. Readers are invited to help stop the stigma associated with mental illness and raise awareness of symptoms, behaviors, words, and actions related to depression and suicide.

Contemporary adolescent literature and mainstream media are beginning to tell more stories about people who struggle with opioid use. Stories about the psychological and emotional impact of opioid use and abuse are especially important for adolescents to explore, as the United States faces a national opioid crisis (Department of Health and Human Services [HHS], 2019). Amanda Rigell, Arianna Banack, and Allen Rigell's chapter provides teachers information and strategies to guide students through narratives about opioid abuse, scaffold students' research skills, and help them become more informed about our national health crisis through a reading of Mindy McGinnis's (2019) novel, *Heroine*. The instructional strategies featured within this chapter aim to assist teachers as they seek to strengthen students' ability to make real-world connections through research and intertextual connections.

Caitlin Corrieri and Elyana Genovese take readers on a hero's journey into the world of obsessive-compulsive disorder (OCD) as experienced by the protagonist of Wesley King's (2016) middle-level novel, *OCDaniel*. This chapter provides teachers a means of expanding students' mental health literacy while building their understanding of the hero's journey theme as they follow Daniel, the protagonist of the novel, on his voyage of self-discovery and acceptance. The activities featured throughout the chapter encourage students to practice empathy by taking the perspectives of various characters as they examine those characters' conflicts and decisions, challenge stigma and stereotypes around mental illness, and engage with Daniel's journey as one of self-discovery, courage, and strength: the true marks of a hero.

Our final chapter offers teachers guidance and suggestions regarding ways they can utilize book clubs to foster mental health literacy through adolescent fiction. Lesley Roessing and Jessica Traylor provide teachers detailed suggestions for implementing book clubs in the classroom using five specific novels that cover a variety of mental health concerns: *Scars* by Cheryl Rainfield (2010), *Saving Red* by Sonya Sones (2016), *Wintergirls* by Laurie Halse Anderson (2009), *The Unlikely Hero of Room 13B* by Teresa Toten (2013), and *The Memory of Light* by Francisco X. Stork (2017). Teachers can choose to implement book clubs without additional preparation if they choose one or more of the suggested novels. Roessing and Traylor provide a thoughtful and detailed description of the book club process, beginning with allowing students to choose from a limited selection of novels and then engaging in pre-reading lessons on the foundational elements of mental health literacy and reading literacy. Next, teachers are shown how they might model the process of what students are to look for in reference to each of the mental health literacy and reading literacy lessons. The chapter ends with several examples of group projects that can be used in the assessment of book clubs.

CONCLUSION

Within the ensuing pages, educators are provided access points across a variety of books for increasing mental health awareness while attending to ELA content and literacy standards. The notable advantage of this text is located in the coauthorship of an educator and mental health professional featured in each chapter. Their collaborations provide a unique and informative perspective for suggested before-, during-, and after-reading strategies that promote foundational mental health education and ELA competencies and support prosocial action.

REFERENCES

Ali, D. (2017). *NASPA policy and practice series: Safe space and brave spaces; Historical context and recommendation for student affairs professionals* (Policy Brief No. 2). Washington, DC: National Association of Student Personnel Administrators. https://www.naspa.org/images/uploads/main/Policy_ and_Practice_No_2_Safe_Brave_Spaces.pdf

Anderson, L. H. (2009). *Wintergirls*. New York: Viking Books for Young Readers.

Arao, B., & Clemens, K. (2013). From safe spaces to brave spaces: A new way to frame dialogue around diversity and social justice. In L. Landreman (Ed.), *The art of effective facilitation: Reflections from social justice educators* (pp. 135–50). Sterling, VA: Stylus.

Aziz, J., Wilder, P., & Mora, R. A. (2019). YAL as a tool for healing and critical consciousness. *ALAN Review, 46*(2), 71–78.

Casey, B. J., & Caudle, K. (2013). The teenage brain: Self control. *Current Directions in Psychological Science, 22*(2), 82–87. https://doi.org/10.1177/0963721413480170

Colorado Senate Bill 18-272. (2019). https://statebillinfo.com/SBI/index.cfm?fuseaction=Public.Dossier&id=24633&pk=736&style=pinstripe

Corrigan, P. W., Morris, S. B., Michaels, P. J., Rafacz, J. D., & Rüsch, N. (2012). Challenging the public stigma of mental illness: A meta-analysis of outcome studies. *Psychiatric Services, 63*(10), 963–73. https://doi.org/10.1176/appi.ps.201100529

Deighton, J., Humphrey, N., Belsky, J., Boehnke, J., Vostanis, P., & Patalay, P. (2018). Longitudinal pathways between mental health difficulties and academic performance during middle childhood and early adolescence. *British Journal of Developmental Psychology, 36*(1), 110–26. https://doi.org/10.1111/bjdp.12218

Department of Health and Human Services. (2019). *What is the U.S. opioid epidemic?* https://www.hhs.gov/opioids/about-the-epidemic/index.html

Florida Department of Education. (2019, July). *Commissioner of Education announces enhanced mental health requirements for Florida schools.* http://www.fldoe.org/newsroom/latest-news/commissioner-of-education-announces-enhanced-mental-health-requirements-for-florida-schools.stml

Hall, M. (2020). Bibliotherapy and OCD: The case of *Turtles all the way down* by John Green (2017). *New Horizons in English Studies, 5*(1), 74–87. http://dx.doi.org/10.17951/nh.2020.5.74-87

Jorm, A. F. (2000). Mental health literacy: Public knowledge and beliefs about mental disorders. *British Journal of Psychiatry, 177*(5), 396–401.

King, W. (2016). *OCDaniel*. New York: Simon & Schuster.

Krosoczka, J. (2018). *Hey, kiddo*. New York: Graphix.

Lake, P. K., Hass, B. K., & Matthews, M. (2014). Fit to care: An action research study exploring the use of Communication Theory to strengthen caring relationships between teachers and students. *International Journal for Human Caring, 18*(3), 15–25. http://dx.doi.org/10.20467/1091-5710-18.3.15

McGinnis, M. (2019). *Heroine*. New York: Katherine Tegen Books.

McLeod, J. D., Uemura, R., & Rohrman, S. (2012). Adolescent mental health, behavior problems, and academic achievement. *Journal of Health and Social Behavior*, 53(4), 482–97. https://doi.org/10.1177/0022146512462888

Merikangas, K. R., He, J. P., Burstein, M., Swanson, S. A., Avenevoli, S., Cui, L., & Swendsen, J. (2010). Lifetime prevalence of mental disorders in US adolescents: Results from the National Comorbidity Survey Replication–Adolescent Supplement (NCS-A). *Journal of the American Academy of Child & Adolescent Psychiatry*, 49(10), 980–89. https://doi.org/10.1016/j.jaac.2010.05.017

Milin, R., Kutcher, S., Lewis, S. P., Walker, S., Wei, Y., Ferrill, N., & Armstrong, M. A. (2016). Impact of a mental health curriculum on knowledge and stigma among high school students: A randomized controlled trial. *Journal of the American Academy of Child & Adolescent Psychiatry*, 55(5), 383–91. https://doi.org/10.1016/j.jaac.2016.02.018

Montgomery, P., & Maunders, K. (2015). The effectiveness of creative bibliotherapy for internalizing, externalizing, and prosocial behaviors in children: A systematic review. *Children and Youth Services Review*, 55, 37–47. https://doi.org/10.1016/j.childyouth.2015.05.010

Moore, A., & Begoray, D. (2017). "The Last Block of Ice": Trauma literature in the high school classroom. *Journal of Adolescent & Adult Literacy*, 61(2), 173–81. https://doi.org/10.1002/jaal.674

Moses, T. (2010). Being treated differently: Stigma experiences with family, peers, and school staff among adolescents with mental health disorders. *Social Science & Medicine*, 70(7), 985–93. https://doi.org/10.1016/j.socscimed.2009.12.022

National Alliance on Mental Illness. (2021). *Mental health by the numbers.* https://www.nami.org/mhstats

Nevada Senate Bill 204. (2019). https://www.leg.state.nv.us/App/NELIS/REL/80th2019/Bill/6348/Overview

O'Driscoll, C., Heary, C., Hennessy, E., & McKeague, L. (2012). Explicit and implicit stigma towards peers with mental health problems in childhood and adolescence. *Journal of Child Psychology and Psychiatry*, 53(10), 1054–62. https://doi.org/10.1111/j.1469-7610.2012.02580.x

Owusu-Ansah, A., & Kyei-Blankson, L. (2016). Going back to the basics. Demonstrating care, connectedness, and a pedagogy of relationship in education. *World Journal of Education*, 6(3), 1–9. https://doi.org/10.5430/wje.v6n3p1

Petro-Roy, J. (2019). *Good enough.* New York: Square Fish.

Rainfield, C. (2010). *Scars.* Lodi, NJ: WestSide Books.

Range, B., Carnes-Holt, K., & Bruce, M. A. (2013). Engaging middle grade students to learn in a caring community. *Clearing House: A Journal of Edu-*

cational Strategies, Issues and Ideas, 86(2), 48–52. htttps://doi.org/10.1080/0 0098655.2012.738438

Reynolds, J. (2015). *The boy in the black suit*. New York: Atheneum Books for Young Readers.

Richmond, K. J. (2014). Using literature to confront the stigma of mental illness, teach empathy, and break stereotypes. *Language Arts Journal of Michigan*, *30*(1), 6. https://doi.org/10.9707/2168-149X.2038

Richmond, K. J. (2019). *Mental illness in young adult literature: Exploring real struggles through fictional characters*. Santa Barbara, CA: ABC-CLIO / Libraries Unlimited.

Rodriguez, C. L. (2015). *When Reason Breaks*. New York: Bloomsbury.

Rogers, C. R. (1961). *On becoming a person*. Boston, MA: Houghton Mifflin.

Rosenblatt, L. M. (2005). *Making meaning with texts*. Westport, CT: Heinemann.

Russell, K. (2019). *A sky for us alone*. New York: Katherine Tegen Books.

Sánchez, E. L. (2017). *I am not your perfect Mexican daughter*. New York: Knopf.

Sones, S. (2016). *Saving Red*. New York: HarperTeen.

Stork, F. (2017). *The memory of light*. Arthur A. Levine.

Substance Abuse and Mental Health Services Administration. (2014). *SAMHSA's Concept of trauma and guidance for a trauma-informed approach* (HHS Publication No. 14-4884). http://store.samhsa.gov/shin/content/SMA14-4884/ SMA14- 4884.pdf

Texas House Bill 18 (2019). https://legiscan.com/TX/bill/HB18/2019

Toten, T. (2013). *The unlikely hero of room 13B*. Toronto: Doubleday Canada.

Vestal, C. (2018, June 23). *States begin requiring mental health education in schools*. National Alliance on Mental Illness Virginia. https://namivirginia .org/states-begin-requiring-mental-health-education-schools/

Zhao, W., Young, R. E., Breslow, L., Michel, N. M., Flett, G. L., & Goldberg, J. O. (2015). Attachment style, relationship factors, and mental health stigma among adolescents. *Canadian Journal of Behavioural Science/ Revue Canadienne des Sciences du Comportement*, *47*(4), 263. https://doi .org/10.1037/cbs0000018

WHAT'S MINED IS OURS

Mental Health and American Rurality in Kristin Russell's *A Sky for Us Alone*

Jeff Spanke and Sara Tyner

We've all seen the movie before. A well-to-do family is enjoying their quiet, peaceful, painless life in the suburbs. Just when all the rightness of the world solidifies in a perfectly cooked turkey and a fine French wine, the bad guys show up and wreak havoc on the otherwise tranquil abode. Panic ensues, threats are made, special forces are called in. There's a briefcase with a digital lock and a hidden safe, and Bruce Willis plays the hero.

In the end, of course, the bad guys lose. Windows break, stained shirts get ripped, and just as the sun starts to rise over the horizon after a long night in hell, the shot widens to an overhead of our hero escorting the family—all huddled together, cloaked in fleece blankets and limping—to the squad cars lining the perimeter, lights blinking, sirens singing. Roll credits.

We never see the kids go back to school. Nor, for that matter, do we ever see the windows get fixed, the furniture replaced, the blood mopped from the hardwood or sopped from the carpet. The story's victory lies in these characters surviving the traumatic event itself, as if suffering and pain are finite, singular enterprises flanked on both sides by the arrival and departure of bad.

The thing is, of course, these kids will still have nightmares. And any semblance of the parents' normality will forever remain splattered among the shattered remnants of "that night." Yet, even though it never makes the final cut, the affluent status of the family will likely afford these victims bountiful resources to treat their various mental and physical needs long after the final ambulance leaves and the jaded detective closes his latest case.

But what about other families, the ones who don't live in the suburbs? What about the ones who live in the mountains, not as an arboreal respite from the hustle of sub/urban privilege, but because they've just always lived in the mountains? Or on the farm or in the desert? What about the traumas that don't stem from "bad guys" trying to crack a vault or hack into an overseas account but, rather, metastasize through years of poverty, loss, or abuse? What about those families and those kids who can't afford therapy, don't have access to sustained medical care, hunt their own turkeys, or live just far enough off Bruce Willis's radar that their stories never make it to a theater near us?

UNDERSTANDING AMERICAN RURALITY AND MENTAL HEALTH

Indeed, while the fictional families in these films certainly experience their fair share of traumas, large swaths of the American populous often face their own equally paralyzing but uniquely compromising encounters. In fact, Snell-Rood et al. (2017) contend that regional disparities and variations to treatment use and efficacy highlight a crucial need for mental health literacy in rural areas specifically. Crowe et al. (2019) noted that the roughly 90 million U.S. citizens residing in rural populations "must travel greater distances for mental health services, are less likely to have health insurance, and have lower mental health literacy" (p. 382). Smalley et al. (2012) suggest that rural residents may be particularly vulnerable to false or misleading information about mental health disorders because of salient mental health stigmas, a pervasive cultural primacy on self-reliance and autonomy to alleviate mental health concerns, and cultivating perceptions of mental health based on information derived from nonprofessionals.

While young adult literature, as a genre, has a vast tradition of depicting various adolescent traumas, one cultural context that consistently gets marginalized in these narratives is the American rural. One book that succeeds in showcasing the mental health struggles of people living in American rurality is Kristin Russell's (2019) *A Sky for Us Alone*. Through rooting her fictional narrative in the isolated constrictions of the Appalachian region, Russell highlights the extent to which rural adolescents oftentimes lack the language, resources, and cultural support to cope with their situations.

This chapter examines how the rural teen characters in Russell's literary landscape struggle with specific mental health issues and, by extension, highlight the needs of millions of Americans who may not believe there's life outside the coal mines. Additionally, while *A Sky for Us Alone* certainly lends itself well to lessons on several elements of English language arts (ELA), this chapter approaches this text through an ELA lens of character, symbols, and setting. The activities and discussion that follow seek to demonstrate how these literary elements augment the mental health issues of grief, addiction, trauma, and parentification present in the American rural.

A SKY FOR US ALONE BY KRISTIN RUSSELL

In the isolated independence of Appalachia, Kristin Russell anchors her tragic story of Harlowe, a working-class miner's son whose 18th birthday is rocked by the mysterious murder of his older brother, Nate. A literal valley flanks Harlowe's world; below his feet run the countless miles of coal mines. Nate's murder puts into motion a series of tragedies and pitfalls that set Harlowe on an isolated and perilous journey for truth and salvation while ultimately confirming for him what he spent his childhood denying. Yet, despite the futility of Strickland and the damning reality of his impoverished, mine-dwelling future, he meets Tennessee, the beautiful stranger who also knows sadness, loss, and numbness.

GUIDING STUDENTS INTO THE TEXT

Mental Health Literacy and the American Rural

Before readers begin exploring the various symbols buried in and around Russell's story, it's important to develop a working understanding

of the setting of the novel, as well as the specific mental health afflictions faced by its characters. Russell's text depicts mental health
in distinct but inherently linked ways. Following are some key terms
that speak to the mental health and rural themes prevalent within and
throughout the novel.

- *Parentification:* This term refers to "the subjective distortion of the
  relationship as if one's . . . child [were] his parent" (Boszormanyi-
  Nagy & Spark, 1981, p. 151). Caregiving patterns can replace age-
  appropriate social activities and, throughout time, may interfere
  with social and emotional development. Kids become parents to
  their own moms and dads, which means they're simultaneously
  stripped of a childhood *and* thrown into a role for which they are
  in no way equipped and receive no support. Burt (1992) finds that
  childhood parentification often correlates with reports of child
  abuse, and several studies have discovered a connection between
  parentification and alcohol abuse (Burnett et al., 2006; Carroll &
  Robinson, 2000; Chase et al., 1998).
- *Grief:* Kessler (2019) argues that grief occurs internally and should
  be witnessed and acknowledged by others, stating, "The internal
  work of grief is a process, a journey . . . it does not have prescribed
  dimensions and does not end on a certain date" (p. 31). At the
  beginning of the novel, Nate's death precipitates the grief that anchors much of the characters' actions and persists throughout the
  entirety of the narrative.
- *Addiction:* Sussman and Sussman (2011) report that addiction is
  composed of five elements: behaving in a way to achieve appeti-
  tive effects, perseverance on that particular behavior, momentary
  satisfaction, loss of control, and suffering negative consequences.
  Furthermore, just as grief manifests internally, Mate (2010) posits
  that all addictions—"whether to drugs or to non-drug behaviors—
  share the same brain circuits and brain chemicals. On the biochemical level the purpose of all addictions is to create an altered
  physiological state in the brain. This can be achieved in many ways,
  drug taking being the most direct. So an addiction is never purely
  'psychological'; all addictions have a biological dimension" (p. 34).

- *Trauma:* Van der Kolk (2015) notes that "trauma results in a fundamental reorganization of the way mind and brain manage perceptions. It changes not only how we think and what we think about, but also our very capacity to think" (p. 21). The prevailing issue of addiction (drugs and alcohol), as well as the trauma that causes and results from this addiction, really underscores the characters' mental health issues throughout the novel. In this sense, each affliction functions as integral components to the same vicious, generational cycle. Trauma leads to grief, which leads to addiction, which leads to parentification, which leads to more trauma, which breeds upon itself.

Introducing Rurality through Media: A Multimodal Synthesis of Setting

Given the unique cultural backdrop of Russell's American rurality, students should understand that Harlowe's approach to a life plagued by trauma and grief differs significantly from the way an urban or suburban teen with access to mental health treatments (and community support to seek such care) may cope with their circumstance. To prepare students to read a novel set in a particular region of the rural United States, as well as to guide students in their reading, teachers could take time to offer multimodal representations of that context. Table 1.1 provides

Table 1.1. Multimodal Depictions of American Rurality

Nonfiction	Film Trailers	Photographers	Other Media
Selected excerpts from the following:	*Troop Zero* (2019)	Rich-Joseph Facun	"Blackberry Motorist" by Richard Brautigan
Hillbilly Elegy (2018)	*Three Billboards Outside Ebbing, Missouri* (2017)	Miles Orvell	"Sticks" by George Saunders
Appalachian Reckoning (2019)	*Wind River* (2017)	Tema Stauffer	"A&P" by John Updike
What We're Getting Wrong about Appalachia (2018)	*Hell or High Water* (2016)	Todd Hido	"The Lottery" by Shirley Jackson
Appalachian Fall (2020)	*No Country for Old Men* (2007)	John Horvath	"The Split Cherry Tree" by Jesse Stuart
Soul Full of Coal Dust (2020)	*Gummo* (1997)	Seph Lawless	
	Deliverance (1972)	Gregory Crewdson	

some examples of potential media that teachers can use to further contextualize American rurality prior to beginning the text. Justifications and possible applications of these media are offered below.

Nonfiction

To avoid framing rurality in terms of stereotypes or antiquated/inaccurate assumptions, teachers could first contextualize Russell's novel through the incorporation of nonfiction media. This can include contemporary essays, memoirs, or credible news articles, as well as shorter historical texts of similar nature. In addition to addressing student learning objectives that stress the curricular inclusion of various nonfiction texts, the use of this material will also help students operationally conceive of rurality as a real phenomenon experienced by real people throughout the vast United States. Additionally, teachers can use these texts to explore problematic or reductive representations of rurality—*Hillbilly Elegy*, for example—within nonfiction media.

Film Trailers

Having begun the process of developing informed views of rural populations, teachers may also want to augment their pre-reading with examples of cinematic representations of American rurality. More often than not, when American rurality is featured in cinema, it is done so through a lens of either fear or ridicule—that is, both the region itself and the citizens therein function as scary things where people vanish or die, or as things simply to make fun of. As singular multimodal ensembles in themselves, film trailers make wonderful additions to the English language arts classroom because they require virtually no outside context, their content has typically been approved for wide audiences, and their short length and unique rhetorical construction make them ideal tools for quick, efficient narrative exposure. Through using rural film trailers, students can analyze and synthesize common thematic elements of rural representation, as well as dispel salient stereotypes and misconceptions by juxtaposing the trailers with the nonfiction material they studied earlier. With film trailers, teachers can engage students

in critical explorations not of the plots of the individual movies themselves but, rather, how those plots and depictions of rurality speak to
the greater conditions of poverty, disenfranchisement, and isolation in
these populations. How do these trailers contribute to the dominant
narrative of American rurality, and what limitations and/or affordances
operate in that cinematic contribution? What values do they confirm?
Which do they challenge?

Photographs

   In keeping with the realm of the aesthetic, photographs and other
still images offer students an illustrative means to engage with rurality
in ways that exceed the parameters of printed text. Photo series, paint-
ings, and advertisements can offer a perspective of rurality that can't
be achieved through other modalities. Photo series, in particular, can
imbue the critical study of rurality with a narrative style that demands
more of students than film trailers, news videos, or documentaries. With
photographs, students must rely on not only the analytic and synthesizing skills that characterize how they read other types of texts, but also,
and perhaps more important, the various visual and rhetorical skills
needed to navigate as critically thinking citizens. The unique vision that
students cultivate through engaging with photographs and other visual
art can help punctuate an already burgeoning understanding of American rurality as both space and place.

Other Media

   What makes film trailers, photographs, and essays conducive to productive scaffolding is the fact they all demand very little in terms of
time, preparation, or contextualization. Each of these media lend themselves to a variety of teaching strategies and student learning styles—
from lectures and presentations to small-group work and multimodal,
individual student composition. Adding to this list of multimodal representations of rurality are other media such as short stories and musical
compositions. With this material, again, teachers can take advantage of
their short length and accessibility.

Making Sense of the Media

Because of the volume of contextual material available for readers prior to engaging in the novel, teachers should be deliberate and intentional with how they employ these materials, especially to avoid stereotyping or somehow othering residents of these regions or the regions themselves. Teachers could show the film trailers, for example, with an exclusive attention on "mood," inviting students to analyze the various feelings and affective appeals of these rural depictions. In this case, students would view and study the trailers as unique texts in themselves, analyzing them for the respective compositional elements that create the mood, as opposed to using the trailers to analyze or "diagnose" broader elements of American rurality. The focus, then, would be on the mood of the *trailer*, not the students' judgment of the *rural*.

This could be in conjunction with analysis of the photographs through a lens of "light" or "space," in which students document how the artists use space in the images to convey a particular theme. The more literary media could be used as springboards to engage with "character" or "plot," the more opportunity for nonfiction sources to be approached with a focus on conflict or tension. As teachers share these materials, the students could keep a written account of the various elements of their focus—theme, mood, tensions, and characters, for example—that teachers could then use to help students form conclusions, predictions, and even further questions about what they're about to read.

No matter the specific use of the media, each medium can be used to analyze/chart/chronicle or somehow engage with *one* literary element so as not to overwhelm the students or unnecessarily complicate this pre-reading stage. As students compile their potential lists of themes, moods, tensions, spaces, and characters, teachers can then ask them to start comparing their data, finding similarities and gaps in their findings.

ELA Applications: The Flags We Carry

After teachers offer some background on rurality and introduce terminology and definitions on the mental health issues prevalent in the text (addiction, grief, trauma, and parentification), and before students begin reading the novel, teachers can offer some framework for the overarching literary features in the narrative. For students to recognize and understand Russell's depiction of mental health and rurality, it's important for them to be familiar with the figurative language element of symbolism, as well as the literary elements of character and setting.

There are certainly many ways to teach symbolism creatively and effectively. The cultural and visible nature of symbols make them particularly amenable to students who may be more artistically inclined. One way for teachers to introduce/reinforce the concept of symbolism for *A Sky for Us Alone* would be to present a variety of widely known public symbols for students to discuss and deconstruct. Social media logos, professional sports emblems, road signs, and other popular product brands could all be presented to students as the introduction to an activity in which they generate a list of values, traits, and/or characteristics of each image.

Teachers could make a point to explain that symbols are most often public and recognizable; they can change throughout time (as is the case, for example, with the American flag), and their "meaning" often reflects the society that created it and in which it operates. Symbols can have both negative and positive connotations; often operate with varying degrees of power and social capital; and can represent more accessible, objective things like a type of soda or model of car, as well as more grand, abstract concepts like freedom, liberty, and oppression.

A culminating activity for this portion of the pre-reading stage could involve inviting students to create, without words, some sort of symbolic representation (a flag, a logo, a unique image) of the American rural, based on the data derived in the multimodal exercise, that they will display publicly for the duration of the reading. As discussed later in the chapter, since so many of the symbols in Russell's text relate directly to the characters and their setting, it would be important for students to recognize that symbols have a powerful impact on how one sees other people and how one feels about certain places. The symbols that students create should contain images, pictures, and other artistic representations that they feel properly and accurately illustrate whatever aspects of American rurality they wish to showcase. These aesthetic artifacts will later serve as the foundation for the activity that students could complete as they transition away from the text.

GUIDING STUDENTS THROUGH THE TEXT

Exploring Symbolism in the Text

Once students have a clearer image of American rurality and a working knowledge of literary/cultural symbolism, they can begin applying these frameworks directly to the text. *A Sky for Us Alone* contains three overarching symbols prevalent throughout the narrative:

- the mine
- food
- the Ferris wheel

As discussed in the next section, there are certainly other smaller symbols that Russell included in her novel, but the salient symbols of coal mines, food production/consumption, and the Ferris wheel more so serve as mechanisms to tether these characters to each other, their setting, and their respective mental health issues.

In keeping with the emphasis on creative construction and multimodality, teachers can use these literary symbols to invoke further student design and aesthetic projects. For example, in the interest of promoting student agency and choice, teachers could offer the following options for students as they navigate the text. Students could create the following:

Mine Your Own Business

This project combines academic research skills, creativity, and literary analysis. Students begin by conducting research on the coal mining industry, possibly paying specific attention to the particular machinery involved, physical/mental/health risks, economic implications, and cultural/historical traditions. With the findings from this preliminary research at their disposal, students create a chain of (between three and five) "mine cars" that they fill with various symbolic representations of the town of Strickland. Specific questions to guide this construction could include the following:

- What's *really* buried beneath Strickland? What are the treasures below this town? What are the dangers?

- Who are the miners? What are their hopes, dreams? What do they fear? Where do they come from, and where do they go?
- How do the cars *work*? What are they "made of," and why? How has their design changed throughout time? What will they look like in the future, and how will their construction change?

For this exercise, students will construct their cars using whatever materials they choose and, as a way of responding to the previous questions, fill them with various objects, items, and representations of Strickland. The key here, of course, is that every decision the students make— from the material to the items themselves—needs to be grounded in textual evidence and support from the novel. After completing the projects, students will then augment their choices with textual support for their decisions (specific quotations/passages from the text), as well as an explanation for how those bits of evidence justify their claims. In addition to evidence from the novel itself, students should also include information from the research they conducted about the coal mining industry as a means of connecting the fictional Strickland to the real-world tradition of rural coal mining.

Meals Heal the Feels

In addition to the coal mines symbolically representing the town and people of Strickland, food plays an integral symbolic role in *A Sky for Us Alone*. Each of the characters throughout the novel speaks of both the production and consumption of various food items, so much so that food itself ultimately takes on a symbolic representation of pride, power, personhood, and purpose.

For this option, students could design a "Recipes from Strickland" project that operates much like a conventional cookbook. Students could choose a handful (again, maybe between three and five) characters from the novel and compose a series of "recipes" that each character would symbolically make based on the students' analysis of that character. The recipes themselves wouldn't necessarily need to be realistic or even culinarily feasible, of course; the purpose of the activity would be to have students creatively and analytically envision what sort of food a resident of Strickland would produce. And as with a traditional cookbook, the recipes should include "ingredients" and "procedures" for how to prepare the specified item. Of course, this is all under the auspices of symbolism and figurative language.

For example, students may create a recipe for "Harlowe's Birthday Surprise!" The entry for this item may include the following ingredients and steps:

- Start with an apple. Preferably one that fell close to the tree. The more bruised, the better.
- Let it sit for 16 years, keeping it soaked in alcohol. Your choice!
- Add a dash of bitterness and pinch of spite.
- As it ages, sprinkle in some hope.
- Keep it in the sun so it gets tough.
- Be sure to keep the skin on; try to avoid any cracks in the outer layer.
- Expose it to smoke and other chemicals so it loses its color.
- After 16 years, cut it in half and remove its core.
- Dice the hope. Pitch the core. We don't need it.
- Cut up the remaining apple into tiny bits. Bury a few. Eat a few. Throw the rest in a blender and mash.
- When the apple is a mushy pulp, form it into a ball and place it back under the tree where it came from.
- Lick the bowl. And enjoy.

For each step in the recipe, students should include a citation from the text to justify/explain this step in the procedure. Teachers should emphasize that the point of this exercise isn't to judge, condemn, or speculate—nor is it to bake "ourselves" into these recipes—but rather to understand and engage with these characters through the lens of food production and consumption, just as the characters themselves do throughout the novel.

As students compile their recipes and corresponding analyses, they can decorate their cookbooks with images and other symbols that highlight various aspects of the characters and the food item being discussed. The classroom is now becoming a Strickland of its own, with miniature mine cars depicting the town and its residents, and cookbooks made for/by/of our characters.

Ferris Wheel's Day On

While the mines and food are the most prevalent symbols in the novel, one symbol that occupies a relatively short amount of time compared to the other two, but that certainly influences the trajectory of the narrative, is the Ferris wheel. For Harlowe and Tennessee, the Ferris wheel that appears during the county fair represents freedom and liberation, hope and transcendence. It symbolizes their potential to elevate above their circumstance and enlivens their prospect that they don't have to become their parents, and they don't have to die in the mines. Its transient nature, though—the fact that it, as with all fairs, doesn't last long—highlights its fleeting reality.

For this activity, students could create a miniature Ferris wheel that consists of three to five separate cars. Though in contrast to the previously buried secrets that were unearthed by the mining option, this project invites students to fill the cars with the hopes and dreams of the novel's characters. As with the other two options, students could create the Ferris wheel cars in whatever form, using whatever materials they desire, and fill them, again, with items and objects that reflect the dreams of the characters.

And as with the other two options, students should accompany their artistic choices with evidence-based responses that explain these decisions. For example, if a teacher wanted to guide a student in their creation of Tennessee's Ferris wheel car, they could ask:

- What would Tennessee bring with her on her ride? Why?
- What would she want to see at the top of the ride?
- What would she not want to see?
- What would she be thinking as she's going up? Going down?
- How many times would she ride, and who would she ride with?

Again, each of these options position the three prominent symbols in the novel as a catalyst for student close reading, research, analysis, and multimodal compositions. These literacy skills and language functions are funneled through the literary symbols of the mine, food, and the Ferris wheel. The minor symbols of the novel also lend themselves to student analysis and artistic creation and, in doing so, serve as a tether between literacy skills and the mental health issues prevalent in the reading.

Bridging Symbolism to Mental Health

In addition to engaging with the three overarching symbols discussed earlier, one way for students to develop their understanding of some of the more minor symbols operating in the book is through the use of a Literary Identification activity (see table 1.2). This exercise has two components: one analytical, and the other artistic. The key with the first portion of this exercise is that, rather than asking students to respond to an open-ended prompt or explicate an abstract idea or literary motif, teachers could select specific items/artifacts—symbols—from the text and have students use that item to respond to a series of questions. Possible questions could include the following:

1. What *is* the item/artifact?
2. What role does it serve in the book?
3. Why is it significant? What is it a symbol *for?*
4. As you continue reading, how does this artifact inform the plot?
5. Which characters are affected by this and how?
6. What, if any, mental health issue from the American rural is connected to this artifact?

Student responses to this activity serve as a foundation for the exercise that follows. In this section, they're continuing to develop their critical-thinking, close-reading, and literary analysis skills, all integral ELA objectives performed through the lens of symbolism. Having compiled their responses to these questions and properly identified/contextualized these symbols, the students can now apply their thinking to a more multimodal activity.

Table 1.2.   Examples of Literary Identifications in *A Sky for Us Alone*

Yellow Boy	Pills	Sip N Sac	Geode	Kool-Aid
pp. 176, 249	pp. 54, 83, 187	pp. 26, 35, 39	p. 71	p. 174
Heat/Hate	Mermaids	Roots	Pies	Tents
pp. 1, 44, 173	p. 69	p. 65	pp. 51, 141	p. 218
Saw	Chatham	Crystals	Catfish	Shine
pp. 2, 109, 113	pp. 51–53	p. 66	p. 37	p. 221

Mental Health and Acrostic Memes

For this activity, students are blending acrostic poetry with meme creation. An acrostic poem is a poem in which the first letter of every line spells out a word or phrase when placed in sequential order. In this case, students should choose a symbol from table 1.2 (or multiple symbols) and, using their responses from the prior activity as a frame of reference, create an acrostic for that symbol. For example, "Sip N Sac" could become

Sometimes, you get more than you came for.
I know I sure didn't expect to meet anyone that day . . .
Probably because ya don't meet too many people here.
Never anyone as pretty as her, at least.
Still, there she was.
And my life will never be the same.
Could it be that living is actually better than dying?

Once students have composed their acrostic, they can create a series of memes, one meme per letter/line in their acrostic. In essence, the students are compiling a collection of symbols that build upon symbols, that build upon symbols, that all go back to their analysis of a story and its connection to the mental health issues therein. And of course, as with the activities just described, students should provide textual evidence for their acrostics, as well as written justification/explication of the images they chose to construct their meme series.

Finally, since each one of the these symbols connects to at least one of the mental health issues prevalent in the novel in some way, students should explain how their meme series connects to those issues. It's clear that students have tremendous flexibility and agency in each of these projects; in exchange, it's incumbent on them to justify their decisions, not only with textual evidence but also with connections to rurality and notions of trauma, grief, addiction, and parentification.

Discussion Questions

As a means of balancing the mental health foci and the critical close reading, teachers could also blend the reading of the text with discussion questions. The following questions could potentially aid in whole class conversations; small-team workshops; informal, individual student compositions; or potentially even as part of a larger summative assessment

- Early in the book, Harlowe tells us that "almost all of Mama's family was buried out front" (p. 11). After Nate is killed, we learn that Harlowe's community takes burials very seriously, from their preparation to the actual burial itself. What role does tradition play in the novel? What traditions do we have as a community or country? What makes these traditions worth keeping? What do we gain by honoring them? What do we risk? How do rituals pertaining to death/mourning help or hinder the grieving process? How is loss and/or grief processed in the Strickland community?
- We learn that Harlowe's mama used to host a Bible study (p. 34). What role do you think faith plays in the lives of the people of Strickland? What value does it bring them, and what comfort does it offer?
- Throughout the book, Harlowe casually discusses all the people in his life who have died. Yet, he never talks about these people in terms of loss. Is there a difference between feeling lost and experiencing *loss*? Can someone experience a loss but not feel lost? Can someone feel lost without experiencing a sense of loss? Which of these characters have experienced the most loss? Which seem to feel the most lost? What is the connection among feeling, being, and experiencing, and how do we see this connection in Strickland?
- One of Harlowe's main struggles in this book involves him encountering a lot of different secrets in his town. Some of these secrets involve relationships, behaviors, lies, and realities. Why do you believe the people of Strickland keep secrets? What do the citizens gain by doing so? What do they risk? How do the secrets impact the relationships between characters in the novel?
- When Harlowe begins using the saw that Nate gave him for his birthday, he says, "I figured if you're going to sit at that table for most of your life, it should look as good as it is strong" (p. 110). What does strength look like in Harlowe's world? How does this perception of strength speak to "goodness"?
- After Harlowe yells at his mom for taking too many pills, he notes, "she looked at me like a kid that's been scolded. I hated sounding like the parent that done it. The order of things was all messed up"

(p. 156). What does Harlowe mean by "the order of things"? What is the *order* to life in Strickland? What resources does Harlowe have in his life to help maintain this order? Who could he look to for help? In what other ways do Harlowe and Tennessee act as parents in this novel, and what impact do you think that could have on them as they get closer to adulthood?

- At the carnival, Harlowe enjoys a unique perspective of Strickland as he sits on the Ferris wheel. From this height, he imagined life with Omie and Tennessee "away from the Praters, mines, Mama and Daddy" (p. 209). How does his literal change of perspective in this scene alter how he views the world? What can he see from the ride that he couldn't see on the ground?
- Harlowe returns to the mining plant for the first time in years. He notes the difference in the landscape, how the mine has taken over, and how "almost everything else around had been flat-topped" (p. 227). What role does nature play in this book? Not just the mountain, the mines, the rivers, and the ravines, but all of nature?
- Harlowe's victory in this book comes from reconciling the circumstances of his past and taking steps toward crafting his own "chance that I might really live" (p. 319). How do we feel about this conclusion? Is this a healthy move on Harlowe's part? How do you define the phrase *"really live,"* as it pertains to the story?
- What role does addiction play in the novel? What are the sources of addiction, and what are its consequences? We know that Harlowe's mama struggles with and suffers from addiction, but does Harlowe? Is he addicted to anything? What about Tennessee? Are there different forms of addiction in Strickland, and if so, how might each of these characters overcome their specific afflictions with addiction?

GUIDING STUDENTS OUT OF THE TEXT

A Call to Action

Mining Our Characters

In keeping with the spirit of symbolism and analysis, students could conclude their reading of the text by selecting a specific character and, drawing from Russell's use of Strickland's mine-as-symbols for body/ mind, depict the process of "mining" the character. A prominent theme in *A Sky for Us Alone* suggests that, as people, we are all more than the sum of our parts; that our pasts don't define us and that our futures and fate—our *lives*—are ours to create. In this vein, teachers could invite students to mine, dig up, or somehow resurrect or unearth one of the characters in the story.

For example, students could "mine" the character of Tennessee. If readers were to *analyze* Tennessee's character, they may find her to be "docile, non-threatening, accommodating to her surroundings and amenable to various structures/systems being imposed on her. She is a young, relatively unexamined mine guarded by fierce external obstacles but likely yielding vast treasures. Beneath the surface lies a beauty and a compassion; a uniquely nurturing, maternal impulse that allows those around her to flourish. In the rich and uncharted caverns of her mines lie a deep wisdom and culinary acumen; a sharp maternal instinct and social strength; and a survivalist rigor that resists the imposition of the structures above. Access to her mine is limited and treacherous; extraction comes with a cost, as evidenced by the harshness of her father."

But that's just the analysis.

Mining her character demands a materiality that an analysis can't quite provide. Table 1.3 offers suggestions on how to convert a character analysis to a material mining of Tennessee's character. The point here, again, is to visibly demonstrate that the *stuff* that comprises one's identities—the *things* that seemingly define us and "make us" who we are—are precisely that: things. People are all far grander and worth more than whatever stuff gets taken out of and put back into the earth. As the students gather their "ore"—either the real things themselves or images of the things—with the activities outlined here, they should provide textual support for their items, as well as a justification for their inclusion. Ideally, as students would perform this task, the class would be collecting several seemingly useless and arbitrary items. Again, the point here is to be able to, as a class, physically look upon the *stuff* and recognize that, on one hand, it's not just a flashlight, for example; it's really a symbol of Tennessee's inner strength. But on the other hand, Tennessee has so much more to offer the world than any pile of items can ever report.

Table 1.3. Character Analysis and Its Corresponding Material Mining

What an Analysis May Yield: Tennessee is . . .	What Students Could Symbolically "Mine" from the Character Tennessee
Docile, nonthreatening	Rabbit's foot
Accommodating to her surroundings	Belt
Amenable to various structures/systems being imposed on her	Rubber band
Young and relatively unexamined	An egg
Guarded by fierce external obstacles	Keep Out sign
Likely yielding vast treasures	Jewelry box
Beneath the surface lies a beauty and a compassion	Shovel
Uniquely nurturing, maternal impulse that allows those around her to flourish	Bag of seeds
Rich and uncharted caverns	Pennies
Deep wisdom and culinary acumen	Spatula
Survivalist rigor	Compass
Imposition of the structures above	Padlock
Access to her mine is limited/treacherous	Flashlight

Closing the Book

A Sky for Us, All One

Despite its title, very little of *A Sky for Us Alone* actually focuses on the sky, or really even mentions it at all. Yet, something about Harlowe's journey and the epiphany he and Tennessee both have at the conclusion of the story suggests that the sky is not something one can afford to ignore. In the spirit of transitioning from the text (as well as in a vein of victory and empowerment commensurate to Harlowe's final departing triumph), teachers could invite students to share in Harlowe's enlightenment.

As one final act of symbolism and analysis, students could compose their own origin story behind a constellation of their creation. There is but one sky; and in it, nobody should be alone. Just as actual constellations pay homage to some mythical figure, these creative projects invite students to think of themselves as heroes worthy of being mapped in the stars. Questions guiding this exercise could include the following:

- What shape is your constellation? What symbolic form does it take?
- What is the name of your constellation? Where does that name come from?

- What is your triumph? What is your victory?
- Who/what were your adversaries, and how did you overcome them?
- Did you have tools, helpers? Did you have guidance in any way?
- How many stars are in your constellation, and what symbolic names might they have?

Students could compose their constellation stories in narrative form or some other digital multimodal composition, but regardless of mode and form, teachers could provide materials for students to actually plot their constellation in the sky. As students complete the novel and transition from the text, teachers could collect the individual star maps—complete with their origin stories, explanations, and supporting materials—and combine them into one large, vast, class-specific galaxy that may or may not resemble what Harlowe might have seen from the top of that Ferris wheel.

At this point, the classroom has transformed into a community of its own, with mine cars reflecting American rurality, cookbooks that offer recipes for characters, Ferris wheels packed with their hopes and dreams, thematic memes that draw attention to the embedded mental health issues, and a sky above that looks down on everything, filled with the constellations of the student heroes who built the town below

CONCLUSION

People suffer from trauma and addiction in all communities; and, of course, even though a particular region may not traditionally speak of these afflictions or have resources to address them, that doesn't mean they don't exist or that the people therein don't need help. Indeed, Russell imbues her Strickland with a certain universal tension, that of the liberating impulses of valleys and the oppressive mechanization of the mountains that envelop them. Everyone has mines. Their permanence makes them hard to ignore, and their hardness can lead to a permanent ignorance of their toxicity. But the transient nature of the Ferris wheel—constantly packing up and leaving—invites students to seek out those moments of elevation, however fleeting, and those chances to change one's perspective and empathetically gaze upon our collective circumstance with clearer heads, refined vision, and a light on the horizon. From the oppression of our mines, like Harlowe, we too may rise. Bruce Willis would want it that way.

REFERENCES

Boszormenyi-Nagy, I., & Spark, G. M. (1981). *Invisible loyalties*. New York: Brunner/Mazel.

Burt, A. M. (1992). *Generational boundary distortion: Implications for object relations development* (Doctoral dissertation, Georgia State University, 1992).

Burnett, G., Jones, R. A., Bliwise, N. G., & Ross, L. T. (2006). Family unpredictability, parental alcoholism, and the development of parentification. *American Journal of Family Therapy*, 34(3), 181–89. https://doi.org/10.1080/01926180600550437

Carroll, J. J., & Robinson, B. E. (2000). Depression and parentification among adults as related to parental workaholism and alcoholism. *Family Journal—Counseling and Therapy for Couples and Families*, 8(4), 360–67. https://doi.org/10.1177%2F1066480700084005

Chase, N. D., Demin, M. P., & Wells, M. C. (1998). Parentification, parental alcoholism, and academic status among young adults. *American Journal of Family Therapy*, 26(2): 105–14.

Crowe, A., Averett, P., Avent Harris, J. R., Crumb, L., & Littlewood, K. (2019). In my own words: Exploring definitions of mental health in the rural southeastern United States. *Professional Counselor*, 9(4), 381–95. https://doi.org/10.15241/ac.9.4.381.

Kessler, D. (2019). *Finding meaning: The sixth stage of grief*. New York: Scribner.

Maté, G. (2010). *In the realm of hungry ghosts: Close encounters with addiction*. Berkeley, CA: North Atlantic Books.

Mohatt, D. F., Bradley, M. M., Adams, S. J., & Morris, C. D. (2006). *Mental health and rural America: 1994–2005: An overview and annotated bibliography*. Washington, DC: U.S. Department of Health and Human Service, Office of Rural Health Policy.

Russell, K. (2019). *A sky for us alone*. New York: Katherine Tegen Books.

Smalley, K. B., Warren, J. C., & Rainer, J. P. (Eds.). (2012). *Rural mental health: Issues, policies, and best practices*. New York: Springer.

Snell-Rood, C., Hauenstein, E., Leukefeld, C., Feltner, F., Marcum, A., & Schoenberg, N. (2017). Mental health treatment seeking patterns and preferences of Appalachian women with depression. *American Journal of Orthopsychiatry*, 87, 233–41. http://doi.org/10.1037/ort0000193.

Sussman, S., & Sussman, A. N. (2011). Considering the definition of addiction. *International Journal of Environmental Research and Public Health*, 8(10), 4025–38. https://doi.org/10.3390/ijerph8104025

van der Kolk, B. (2015). *The body keeps the score: Brain, mind, and body in the healing of trauma*. New York: Penguin.

②

LITERACY AND LOSS

Examining Loss and Grief through Characterization in *The Boy in the Black Suit*

Sherri Harper Woods and Terry Benton

Losing a loved one in death can be a traumatic experience for anyone, and perhaps even more so for young people. Adolescents can learn about loss, grief, and recovery by reading books about young people who have experienced loss and are going through the grieving process. By paying close attention to the characters in such literature, students can learn to identify types of loss, recognize symptoms of grief, and notice strategies that characters use to cope with their grief, including drawing support from relationships with other characters. As students learn about how characters process grief and their relationships with one another, they can also analyze how characters' traits influence their actions and decisions.

The young adult novel *The Boy in the Black Suit* by Jason Reynolds (2015) can introduce students to the grieving process, the value of peer support, and the utility of structure to help develop social and emotional skills. The novel lends itself to an examination of characterization while enhancing students' mental health literacy concerning loss and the grieving process. In the story, protagonist Matt and his friend Lovey both experience the loss of a close relative. Together, Matt and Lovey mourn their loved ones, experience the stages of grief, and learn about grief support, empathy, and the shared experience of loss. They also come to understand and cope with their feelings as they begin to find meaning in loss and learn to let go of the weight of grief. The following discussion of *The Boy in the Black Suit* will focus on character development and relationships, types of loss, symptoms of grief, and tasks of mourning that aid in grief recovery.

UNDERSTANDING THE GRIEVING PROCESS

The Childhood Bereavement Estimation Model (Burns et al., 2020) estimates that by the age of 18, nearly 7 percent of young people in the United States will lose a close family member to death. In a national poll of bereaved children and teenagers 18 years and under, 75 percent of the respondents reported feeling sad, angry, alone, overwhelmed, and worried. Many of the youths had trouble concentrating on schoolwork, and 41 percent said "they have acted in ways that they knew might not be good for them, either physically, mentally or emotionally" (Siegel, 2012, para. 2). According to Palmer et al. (2016), grieving adolescents tend to prioritize relationships with their peers, centering friendships as an important part of the healing process among this age group. Friendships that develop in the classroom through transformational conversations contribute to the mental and emotional growth of adolescents and can assist them in grief recovery; therefore, it can be beneficial for young people to learn to recognize the symptoms of grief so they can support grieving friends in seeking help from a trusted adult when the grief becomes overwhelming.

Unlike other mental health challenges, everyone experiences loss and grief. Grieving is a natural process and a way of healing and moving forward (Dubi et al., 2017). Grief support can be useful in resolving grief from loss. Reading stories about grieving characters can help students sort through this process, providing a healing space to let go of things that are gone, resolve the grief, and mourn the loss.

THE BOY IN THE BLACK SUIT BY JASON REYNOLDS

Seventeen-year-old Matthew Miller is mourning the loss of his mother to cancer. Overwhelming grief leads Matt's father to alcohol, which makes him emotionally unavailable to his son. When Matt reluctantly accepts employment at a funeral home in his Brooklyn neighborhood, he is surprised to find solace in his new job, where his dress code is a black suit. Matt has always been able to rely on his best friend Chris, and he continues to do so, but he finds additional support in his grief recovery from his new friend Lovey, who is also mourning the death of a loved one, and his boss at the funeral home, Mr. Ray. Throughout the course of the novel, Matt finds a way to process his grief, move forward in his appreciation of life, and take solace in the memories of those he has lost.

GUIDING STUDENTS INTO THE TEXT

Mental Health Literacy: Loss and Grief

The Boy in the Black Suit provides a lens to examine the grieving process and help students gain perspective of loss and grief. Before engaging in reading, students should be introduced to vocabulary and concepts associated with loss and grief. Unless otherwise noted, the following definitions are adapted from Humphrey (2009):

- *Grief:* An emotion generated by an experience of loss and characterized by sorrow and/or distress and the personal and interpersonal experience of loss (throughout the novel).
- *Grief relief:* The adaptive functions, activities, and interventions that assist in managing symptoms of grief (Sausys, 2014, p. 27) (throughout the novel).
- *Grief recovery:* The process of dealing with the emotional shock and disorientation often brought about by death, facing and dealing with the changes and challenges of beliefs about death, and reclaiming and moving on with life (Rich, 2001, p. xviii) (throughout the novel).

- *Loss:* The real or perceived deprivation of something meaningful (throughout the novel).
- *Loss adaptation:* The process of adjusting to loss (chapter 17).
- *Bereavement:* A period of sorrow following the death of a loved one and is always associated with death (throughout the novel).
- *Mourning:* Socially prescribed practices or outward expressions of grief and can apply to both death-related and non-death-related circumstances (throughout the novel).

Types of Loss and Symptoms of Grief

Feelings of loss can occur in response to instances outside of death. Yet, people are not often encouraged to grieve non-death loss. Identifying the types of loss experienced by characters in the text can help students understand the many types of loss and learn to process and work through grief. Losses may be primary or secondary and include the types of loss listed below, which are adapted from Humphrey (2009).

- *Material loss:* Loss of actual physical matter (chapters 11, 12).
- *Role loss:* Loss of a familiar role or function (chapters 3, 9).
- *Relationship loss:* Loss of a particular way of relating with others (throughout the novel).
- *Functional loss:* Loss of use or functioning of a part of one's body (chapters 6, 12).
- *Intrapsychic loss:* Loss within one's own psyche of a way of thinking about oneself, one's future, or the world (chapters 1, 2, 5, 6).

Symptoms of Grief. Matt and other characters in the story experience grief, which is a normal response to loss. Identifying the symptoms of grief can help students become aware of the impact and complex combinations of grief experiences. According to Sausys (2014), grief impacts our mental, emotional, and physical wellness and can also affect us socially. Loss and grief can disrupt every part of our health, especially our mental health.

Mental health symptoms of grief. Grief can affect a bereaved person's ability to think clearly and concentrate. There are other mental health symptoms of grief, too. For example, at the beginning of the story, Matt is offered a job at Mr. Ray's funeral home. As Matt contemplates whether he should accept the job, he worries about having to relive his mother's funeral every day (chapter 1). While it may seem odd, Matt's decision to work at the funeral home and sit in on funerals is his way of retelling the story surrounding the loss of his mother, a mental health symptom of grief. Another mental health symptom of grief is having dreams or images of the deceased. Matt has recurrent dreams of his mother sitting next to him at her funeral (chapters 3, 5, 7, 10).

Emotional symptoms of grief. Throughout the book, Matt experiences sadness, emptiness, and diminished self-concern (chapters 1, 4, 5, 6).

Physical symptoms of grief. These include pain, feeling of tightness in the chest and/or throat, shortness of breath or frequent sighing, fatigue, exhaustion, low energy, sleep pattern disruption (e.g., insomnia or excessive sleep), overeating or anorexia, disruption of cardiac rhythms, digestive system upset, generalized tension, restlessness, irritability, increased sensitivity to stimuli, and dry mouth. For example, upon learning that his dad has been in an accident, Matt feels as though he cannot breathe, and his stomach feels upset (chapters 5, 6).

Social signs of grief. These signs include being isolated from others, withdrawing from social activities, having a diminished desire for social activities, losing friends, and making new friends (Sausys, 2014). When Matt goes back to school after his mother's death, he does not want to be around people, but at other times when he is feeling sad, he feels a strong need to be with his best friend, Chris (chapters 1, 5).

Before-Reading Loss List

To prepare students to discuss the mental health topics of loss and grief as they are presented in the book, teachers can have students brainstorm and document types of loss that can cause grief. The death of a family member or friend is a loss, of course, but there are other types of loss, too. Some examples are a household move, a job loss resulting in a reduction in family income, serious or extended illness of someone in the family, parental divorce or separation, change in the

Table 2.1. Example Pre-reading Loss List

Event	Feeling
Family moves to a different home	Loneliness
Mom loses her job	Fear
Grandma has breast cancer	Anger
Parents get a divorce	Trapped

status of a friendship, or the loss of a beloved possession. Students can work together to identify other losses. Teachers can use this list, and the feelings these losses can provoke, as a basis for discussing loss and grief vocabulary before reading the book. In the pre-reading activity illustrated in table 2.1, students can document a list of losses they, or others, might have experienced and the feelings associated with the losses.

Once students begin reading the novel, they can create a Loss List specific to the book, similar to the one in table 2.4 later in the chapter.

Introducing Characterization

There is not just one type of loss or singular way in which to grieve. Readers can examine loss and grief by analyzing characters and thereby have the opportunity to see how individuals uniquely experience and navigate loss and grief. Authors develop their characters in a variety of ways. As they describe characters' physical appearance, actions, choices, words, thoughts, and emotions, they also reveal each character's personality, experience, and identity formation throughout the course of the novel. Additionally, readers can learn about characters indirectly as they interact with and respond to other characters. In this activity, teachers can prepare students to explore characterization by asking them to do the following:

- Brainstorm a list of characters they have read about in class together or their favorite characters from other books, television shows, movies, or other popular culture;
- Identify what they like (or dislike) about the characters, what adjectives they would use to describe them, and how they have come to know what they know about the characters;
- Select a character and explain how that character might respond to a given situation, describing what characteristics led students to draw this conclusion;

- Choose a different character and explain what actions that character would take in the same situation, describing how the second character's traits might lead them to act differently than the first character.

Based on responses to these prompts, students can use this foundational understanding to document and track character development and the ways in which students approach and engage with the story as they read *The Boy in the Black Suit*.

Chapter Titles

Before beginning to read the novel, teachers can create a list of the chapter titles, similar to the example in table 2.2. Teachers can then ask students to formulate predictions for each chapter based upon each title. Students can compare their predictions with classmates to gain insight into the ways in which others have inferred meaning or understanding as a result of each chapter title. Later, as students read the novel, they can revisit their predictions and document notes about the events of the chapter, analyze the significance of the title based on their newfound understanding of the text, and discuss whether or not they believe the chapter title is appropriate to the context of the novel. Students can also suggest a different title if they believe a different title would be more appropriate or suitable to the content or character development identified within the chapter. After students complete their reading of the book, teachers can have them revisit their initial list of predictions and further analyze, first, the importance of the events in that chapter, and second, the title's significance to the entirety of the book, the characters, and the book's demonstration of loss and grief.

GUIDING STUDENTS THROUGH THE TEXT

Tracking Character Development

Throughout their reading of *The Boy in the Black Suit*, students can analyze the characters, their individual and collective experiences with loss and grief, and the ways in which the characters support one another through their grief. Teachers can pause after every chapter to discuss

Table 2.2. Chapter Title Prediction Example

Chapter Title	Prediction before Reading	After Reading Chapter	After Finishing Book
Chapter 2: Head to Foot	Students write their predictions here	• Matt and Chris live on opposite ends of the same block—Matt in a single-family brownstone, Chris in a multifamily apartment building. There's "always a bunch of mess going on" in and outside Chris's building. • On Valentine's Day when the boys were seven, Matt's parents go out on a date and Matt spends the night with Chris and his mom. • Both boys sleep in Chris's bed, head to foot. • At Matt's urging, the boys disobey one of Chris's mom's house rules and investigate when they hear arguing in the hallway and end up witnessing a murder.	• Although Chris is now 17 years old, he still always gets home before dark to avoid the violence in and around his building. • In chapter 13, Matt learns that the person who was murdered in the hallway outside of Chris's apartment on Valentine's Day when they were seven years old was Lovey's mother.

what the author has revealed about the characters, how the author has revealed this information to the reader, and any loss and grief the characters have experienced in the chapter. Although students can maintain individual notes, it would be helpful to have students collaborate on a class chart similar to table 2.3 for each character. In this way, students can work together to add information to the class chart as they progress in their reading of the novel. Teachers can introduce a chart for each

Table 2.3. Sample Character Chart

Character's Name: Mr. Willie Ray

What do we learn about this character in this chapter?
Chapter 1
- Well known in the neighborhood
- A funeral director who owns Ray's Funeral Home
- Has recovered from cancer twice
- Talks to other people about cancer; distributes cancer pamphlets
- Walks with a limp
- Friends with Matt's parents; talked with Matt's mom about cancer; helped her get in the ambulance for her last trip to the hospital
- Has a sense of humor; jokes with Matt; joked with Matt's parents
- Offers Matt a job
- Has a positive disposition
- Understanding when Matt initially turns down the job at the funeral home; doesn't try to pressure him; keeps the offer open in case Matt changes his mind
- Knows what to do when a customer gets sick in the Cluck Bucket
- Gives the cashier at the Cluck Bucket some cancer pamphlets to give to her grandmother
- Hires Matt to work at the funeral home
- Uses what Matt calls "old-school slang"
- Seems eager to give Matt advice about girls
- Surprised when Matt asks if he could sit in on a funeral; lets Matt borrow his suit jacket so he would look presentable at the funeral; tells Matt to be respectful at the funeral

How does the author reveal this information?
- The story is told entirely from Matt's point of view, so we learn about Mr. Ray through Matt's first-person narration and through dialogue. Matt already knows Mr. Ray from the neighborhood and as a friend of his parents, but Matt gradually learns more about him.

What kind of loss, if any, does the character experience?
- We learn that Mr. Ray has had cancer twice and that he walks with a limp. The author does not elaborate on those details at this point in the story, but they could indicate functional loss that may be explored later.

What symptoms of grief, if any, does the character display?
- None in this chapter

How does this character relate to other characters in this chapter?
- Mr. Ray is well known in the neighborhood and seems to be well liked.
- Mr. Ray seems to be a caring person as evidenced by his volunteering to inform people about cancer and helping Matt's parents get his mother out of the house and into the ambulance. He also paid attention to the sick customer in the Cluck Bucket and made sure that the manager was aware of the situation. Additionally, he was understanding of Matt's reluctance to work at the funeral home. He cares about his customers. If they are unable to provide for the repast, he makes arrangements to get the food and set up the room for them. When Matt asks to attend the first funeral, Mr. Ray makes sure that Matt is presentable and does not disturb the mourners.
- It seems that Matt respects Mr. Ray, as does the staff at the Cluck Bucket.

character as students encounter them in the book and add additional information to the charts at the conclusion of each chapter. Characters who are central to the text and are therefore developed in greater detail include the following:

Matt Miller, the protagonist
Daisy Miller, Matt's recently deceased mother
Jackson Miller, Matt's father
Chris Hayes, Matt's best friend
The girl who works at Cluck Bucket (We do not find out until chapter 7 that this is Love "Lovey" Brown, who eventually becomes Matt's girlfriend.)
Mr. Willie Ray, owner of the funeral home where Matt works

The Cooking Notebook

There are times when an author will use an object within the story to reveal additional information or develop characters in greater detail. In chapter 1, the reader learns that Matt and his mother regularly cooked meals together. Cooking with his mother was important to Matt and a way for mother and son to grow closer to one another. Throughout the story, Matt often thinks about the time he spent cooking with his mother and the moments when she shared her wisdom with him. In chapter 2, the reader learns that Matt's mom was preparing a notebook of recipes interspersed with notes and humorous messages for Matt. This cooking notebook holds significant meaning for Matt. Matt's views of the notebook at various points in the story reflect his changing feelings of grief over the loss of his mother. Teachers can have students track Matt's interactions with the notebook throughout the novel and use these moments in further analyzing Matt's developing character and experience through loss and grief. For example, students can contrast Matt's reaction to the notebook in chapter 2 with the way he reacts to it in chapter 10, and then examine how the presence of the notebook in chapter 16 is related to Matt's emotional growth. After each mention of the notebook, students can add to the character charts (i.e., table 2.3) for Matt and his mother by adding what the cooking notebook reveals about Mrs.

Miller's personality and what readers learn about Matt and his relationship with his mom from her commentary in the notebook.

During-Reading Tracking Charts

During-Reading Loss List

To prepare students to recognize and discuss types of loss in the novel, teachers can have students revisit the Pre-reading Loss List (table 2.1) and identify the types of loss represented in the class list. As the class reads and discusses the novel, they can create a Loss List specific for the book, similar to the example shown in table 2.4.

Throughout the book, Matt experiences role loss as a son to his mother; relationship loss with both of his parents as a family unit; relationship loss with his dad who turns to alcohol to numb the pain of grief; and intrapsychic loss as Matt begins to examine who he is and what his future will be like without his mother. Lovey also experiences role, relationship, and intrapsychic loss when her grandmother dies. Other characters experience varying types of loss. Candy Man, a former professional basketball player, experiences material loss, role loss, and relationship loss as a result of his use and abuse of drugs (chapter 11). Mr. Ray experienced functional loss when an injury ended his collegiate basketball career and ruined his hopes of being drafted into the NBA (chapter 6). Mr. Miller experiences functional loss when a near-fatal accident causes him to temporarily lose the use of his legs and leaves him confined to a rehabilitation center (chapters 5, 6, 10).

Through identifying different examples of types of loss via a Loss List specific to the book, students can gain a better understanding of individual character experiences. This promotes awareness of the nuances of loss and how these different types of loss uniquely manifest.

Table 2.4.   Types of Loss and Examples from *The Boy in the Black Suit*

Type of Loss	Examples
Material loss	Candy Man loses stardom (chapter 11)
Role loss	Matt loses his father as a role model (chapter 3)
Relationship loss	Matt loses his mom (throughout the novel)
Functional loss	Mr. Ray's broken knee (chapter 6)
Interpsychic loss	Matt learns that the world is dangerous inside and outside of the apartment (chapter 2)

Symptoms of Grief

Teachers can prepare students to discuss symptoms of grief by revisiting the mental health literacy section of this chapter and having students fill out a grief chart similar to the one in table 2.5. The class can work together to brainstorm what mental, emotional, physical, and social symptoms of grief might look like. After every chapter in the book, students can add examples of grief symptoms exhibited by characters in the text.

Examining these grief symptoms can provide insight into how grief is experienced across a number of bio-psycho-social domains and its specific influence on characters, their motivations, and their actions.

Table 2.5. Symptoms of Grief

Type of Grief Symptoms	Class-Generated Description	Examples from The Boy in the Black Suit
Mental symptoms of grief	Examples: confusion, inability to concentrate	Matt is unable to concentrate when he returns to school (chapter 1).
Emotional symptoms of grief	Examples: sadness, moodiness	When Matt is alone at home in the middle of the day, he recognizes the absence of house noise and the absence of his mother and father (chapter 2).
Physical symptoms of grief	Examples: upset stomach, shortness of breath, crying	Matt says he feels crazy inside when he views Mr. Ray's pain room. He has to try hard to keep his composure because he feels the pain, too, and wants to cry (chapter 6).
Social symptoms of grief	Examples: wanting to be with certain good friends, isolation from others	Matt does not believe he fits in anywhere. He only feels comfortable at funerals where other people are grieving just like him (throughout the book).

Coping with Grief by Attending Funerals

Matt is initially reluctant to accept the job at the funeral home, but he soon discovers that sitting in on funerals is oddly satisfying and provides relief from his symptoms of grief. When Matt attends funerals, he experiences a sense of "me too," recognizing that others are also experiencing grief. For brief moments, being in the company of others who are grieving provides him with feelings of belonging and acceptance. These experiences relieve some of the pain of his mourning and his feelings of isolation. As students read about the funerals listed in table 2.6, have them write a brief description of each funeral and explain how attending funerals helps Matt process his grief.

Table 2.6.   Funerals Matt Attends

Funeral	Brief Description	Why Is This Funeral Significant to Matt? What Does Matt Learn from This Funeral?
The funeral of Clark "Speed-O" Jameson (chapter 1)	This is the first funeral Matt attends at his new job.	Matt is surprised to discover that he feels oddly satisfied after witnessing the grief of Mr. Jameson's daughter, Rhonda.
The funeral of Nancy Knight (chapter 4)	Nancy Knight is a 19-year-old who unexpectedly dies after an asthma attack.	Matt is surprised to learn that the deceased is so young—only two years older than he is. This makes Matt think about his own mortality. He again experiences satisfaction as he watches Nancy's mother and sister grieve.
Various funerals (chapter 7)	Matt describes several different funerals.	Although there are different types of funerals, Matt discovers that he always gets satisfaction from watching the person closest to the deceased grieve.
The funeral of Gwendolyn Brown (chapter 7)	Gwendolyn Brown is Lovey's grandmother. Matt meets Lovey at this funeral.	This funeral is unique for Matt. For the first time, he does not get his usual satisfaction from watching the person closest to the deceased grieve. The bereaved person at this funeral, Lovey, does not behave the way Matt expects her to. This funeral is also unique because Matt breaks his own self-imposed rule and stays for the repast after the funeral where he finally meets Lovey and has his first real conversation with her.
The funeral of Andre Watson (chapter 17)	Andre Watson is another teenager, the young man who tries to get Lovey's phone number the first time Matt sees her in the Cluck Bucket at the beginning of the story (chapter 1).	This is the last funeral mentioned in the book and the first one where Matt does not get to complete his ritual of watching the bereaved. Lovey interrupts Matt from his ritual, and he exits the church to pay attention to her instead of what's happening inside at the funeral.

As students examine the function of each funeral in furthering Matt's evolving experience and development, teachers can connect their reading of the funeral scenes back to their understanding of characterization. Teachers can have students revisit the character charts (table 2.3) and discuss the ways in which the author uses each funeral to further develop Matt's character as well as the characters directly involved in each experience.

Tasks of Mourning

According to Sausys (2014), there are four tasks of mourning that serve as a road map for the grieving process: accept the reality of the loss, process the pain of grief, adjust to a world without the deceased, and find an enduring connection with the deceased in the midst of embarking on a new life. In light of this, teachers can have students identify textual evidence from the book that demonstrates the ways in which Matt is moving forward in his mourning (see table 2.7).

The during-reading tracking charts described earlier provide a systematic way to follow how loss, grief, coping, and mourning can all take shape in unique ways, supporting the idea that everyone, including characters featured in the book, process and respond to these experiences differently.

Table 2.7. Tasks of Mourning

Tasks of Mourning	Evidence That Matt Is Moving Forward with This Task
Accept the reality of the loss	Matt finds himself alone in the middle of the day and becomes keenly aware that his mom is gone, and although his dad is still alive, he is not available for him either (chapter 9).
Process the pain of grief	Matt's attendance at the funerals provides him with symptoms of relief (chapters 1, 4, 7, 17).
Adjust to a world without the deceased	At the funeral of Andre Watson, Lovey distracts Matt from the "action" of witnessing Andre's mother's grief, and Matt realizes that he doesn't need to rely on funerals to help him cope with his grief anymore (chapter 17).
Find enduring connection with the deceased in the midst of embarking on a new life	Matt is finally able to read the cooking notebook without breaking down from grief and use it to cook again (chapter 16).

Discussion Questions

In addition to pausing between chapters to reflect on character development, teachers can take time to engage students in discussion of key events and aspects of the text that encourage critical thinking and consideration of the novel. Teachers can use the following questions to prompt further discussion of the text.

- In chapter 3, Matt says the song "Dear Mama" by Tupac Shakur became his "bedtime song" after the death of his mother. This song is mentioned repeatedly in the novel (chapters 3, 5, and 7). How does "Dear Mama" help Matt process his grief? Matt last mentions the song in chapter 16. How does this final mention of the song differ from the others?
- How does Matt feel about flowers, and why (chapters 1, 2, 7, 9, 15)? What do you think the author is conveying about Matt by having him react so strongly to flowers?
  - Contrast the way Lovey feels about flowers with the way Matt feels about them (chapter 15). How does Lovey's favorite flower relate to the topics of death, loss, and grief (chapter 15)?

- People grieve differently. How does Lovey's loss and grief experience after the death of her grandmother differ from the way Matt experiences the loss of his mother (chapter 7)? Although grief is highly individualized, what might be some reasons for the different grief experiences of Lovey and Matt (throughout the book)?
- Mr. Ray's vault is very important to him (chapter 6). Why does Mr. Ray choose to show it to Matt when, in more than 30 years, he has not shown it to anyone else? Matt has known Mr. Ray for a long time. How does learning about Mr. Ray's vault change the way Matt views him? What does Matt learn about loss and grief from Mr. Ray and his vault?
- In chapter 6, Mr. Ray contrasts the game of chess with the card game I-DEE-clare War. What life lessons does Mr. Ray relate to each game (chapters 6, 13)?
- The story is told entirely through Matt's point of view, so the reader only knows what Matt knows about other characters as Matt learns it. In what ways does this perspective disrupt the reader's

knowledge of Lovey's character? How does the author's decision to reveal the story in this way create suspense about Lovey for the reader (chapters 7, 11, 12)?

- After reading chapter 3, contrast the way Matt chooses to dress with the way his father dresses. What can readers infer about each character by his clothing, and how are their clothing choices related to grief?
- In what ways does the author reveal that Mrs. Miller had a sense of humor (throughout the book)?
- Matt is more than just a "boy whose mother died." What else is going on with Matt? What else do we know about him, and how do we know it (throughout the book)?

GUIDING STUDENTS OUT OF THE TEXT

A Call to Action

Both/And Artwork

In chapter 8, Matt meets Lovey and begins to experience joy in the midst of his sorrow. Teachers can have students explore the concept of both/and instead of the either/or of loss, grief, and sorrow. Teachers can challenge students to use what they have learned about Matt to identify and create a list of things that Matt can be grateful for even though he is grieving. For example, Matt and Chris walking to the bus in the rain and joking with one another in chapter 3, or Matt and Lovey enjoying their time together at the Botanic Garden in chapter 15. Students can extend this activity beyond Matt's experiences and produce a mural of opposites that can exist at the same time, such as joy and sorrow. Students can draw representations on paper and put them together to create this class mural.

Closing the Book

Throughout the story, Matt struggles to cope with his feelings of grief after the loss of his mother. He finds comfort in his friendships with

Table 2.8. Partial Supportive Behaviors and Actions Chart

Examples from the Book	Supportive Behaviors and Actions
Matt feels disconnected socially because his classmates avoid him (chapter 1).	Acknowledge others who may be experiencing grief; don't ignore them.
Matt says he wants Chris to "hold me down and treat me normal just because we had so much history" (chapter 2).	Help provide friends with normalcy.

Chris and Lovey, and he gets support and guidance from a trusted adult, Mr. Ray. Matt also uses his attendance at funerals to help him deal with his grief. Since friends are so important to grieving adolescents (Palmer et al., 2016), it would be beneficial for teachers to have students think about ways young people can be supportive to others who are grieving. Students can identify positive and negative examples of peer interactions from the book and use the noted examples to consider behaviors and actions of support.

Table 2.8 is an example chart of the ways in which students can begin to think about transitioning represented moments of loss and grief in the book into real-life prosocial behaviors. Engaging students in this reflective activity will support their learning and meaning making in better applying mental health literacy beyond the classroom's walls.

CONCLUSION

Unfortunately, everyone will experience loss in some form. By spending time examining and getting to know the characters in *The Boy in the Black Suit*, students can learn about loss and grief, friendship, and recovery. Analyzing, discussing, and writing about the characters, the types of losses they experience, their symptoms of grief, and how they process the pain of their grief can help students understand these mental health issues.

The characters in *The Boy in the Black Suit* care for one another and provide needed support to help their friends deal with their losses. Examining how the author uses characterization in *The Boy in the Black Suit* can help students notice details about characters and strategies authors use to reveal those details in other novels.

REFERENCES

Burns, M., Griese, B., King, S., & Talmi, A. (2020). Childhood bereavement: Understanding prevalence and related adversity in the United States. *American Journal of Orthopsychiatry*, 90, 391–405. https://dx.doi.org/10.1037/ort0000442

Dubi, M., Powell, P., & Gentry, J. E. (2017). *Trauma, PTSD, grief and loss: The 10 core competencies for evidence-based treatment.* Eau Clair, WI: PESI.

Humphrey, K. M. (2009). *Counseling strategies for loss and grief.* Alexandria, VA: American Counseling Association.

Palmer, M., Saviet, M., & Tourish, J. (2016). Understanding and supporting grieving adolescents and young adults. *Pediatric Nursing*, 42(6), 275–81.

Reynolds, J. (2015). *The boy in the black suit.* New York: Atheneum Books for Young Readers.

Rich, P. (2001). *Grief counseling homework planner.* New York: Wiley.

Sausys, A. (2014). *Yoga for grief relief: Simple practices for transforming grieving mind & body.* Oakland, CA: New Harbinger Publications.

Siegel, L. (2012, March 15). New York Life/NAGC conduct first-ever poll of grieving kids. *Business Wire.* https://www.businesswire.com/news/home/20120315005812/en/New-York-LifeNAGC-Conduct-First-Ever-Poll-of-Grieving-Kids

3

FIRST-PERSON PERSPECTIVE

Understanding Adolescent Eating Disorders through *Good Enough*

Laura L. Wood, MaryBeth DeGennaro, and Brooke Eisenbach

Beginning in middle school, there is a significant shift in adolescent body dissatisfaction that has been noted as a precursor to the development of disordered eating (a disturbance in eating patterns not meeting a formal diagnosis) or an eating disorder (Bucchianeri et al., 2013). Furthermore, the $42.9 billion beauty industry (Ridder, 2020) and the rise of social media platforms have been identified as contributors to the onset of disordered eating in adolescents (Marengo et al., 2018).

Eating disorders and body image can be difficult topics to approach, especially because it requires educators to challenge their own assumptions about food, body image, and size. Furthermore, schools may have programming or messaging that is inherently fat-phobic because of the significant negative cultural meanings attached to large bodies in the United States (Clare et al., 2015). When we have the courage to challenge these assumptions and foster an environment that deems all bodies as worthy, we not only offer a preventative environment for eating disorders, but also dismantle oppressive structures.

This chapter focuses on the middle-level novel *Good Enough* by Jen Petro-Roy (2019). Teachers can use this novel in the classroom as a means of safely exploring the topic of eating disorders and body image in service of mental health literacy while engaging learners in exploring the author's development of character and use of metaphor and simile. The book uses first-person narrative journaling to provide the reader a meaningful and relatable look into the thoughts and feelings of the 12-year-old protagonist, Riley, as she works through questions around her eating disorder, body image, and sense of self-worth.

UNDERSTANDING EATING DISORDERS

There are three primary types of eating disorders discussed in the book: anorexia nervosa, involving extreme restriction of food; bulimia nervosa, in which a person engages in cycles of binging and purging; and binge eating disorder, which is when a person consumes significant amounts of food usually in a disconnected and quick fashion, with no purging (American Psychiatric Association [APA], 2013).

An eating disorder can be understood as a protective behavior. As the concept of superheroes and origin stories is particularly accessible to middle school students, a potentially useful metaphor to describe this protective function to middle-level students is by comparing it to a *misguided* hero that arrived to help someone cope (Schwartz & Sweezy, 2019). Usually when an adolescent seeks treatment it is because the eating disorder is no longer working as a coping strategy and the eating disorder behaviors have taken over someone's life to the point that they cannot function well without additional support (Wood, 2015). Eating disorders may often be co-diagnosed with anxiety, depression, or post-traumatic stress disorder. For example, if someone has intense anxiety over academic performance in school and/or perceptions of peers, controlling their food intake or numbing themselves with large portions of food may help regulate the emerging anxious feelings.

Additionally, because we live in a society that profits from unrealistic beauty standards, breaking down such messages and providing new ways to approach the sociocultural aspects of an eating disorder/ disordered eating is crucial (Mills et al., 2017). The Health at Every Size (HAES) Model (Bacon, 2010) provides a framework that can aid teachers in talking about food- or body-related issues with students. The HAES principles are the following: (1) respect, (2) critical awareness, and (3) compassionate care. Teachers incorporating these principles in the classroom can use the HAES model to raise awareness and support discussions about how all bodies, no matter what size, deserve respect and compassion. When we embrace the HAES principles, we can honor differences and make for better spaces for all people in our classrooms and communities.

Good Enough is an ideal text for students to develop an understanding of eating disorders and how body image issues develop. Not only does it offer an accurate portrayal of eating disorder treatment, but through journaling, the novel provides a first-person perspective of the protagonist's complex thoughts and feelings so that the reader may better understand her actions.

GOOD ENOUGH BY JEN PETRO-ROY

Riley is a "normal" and happy 12-year-old—that is, until a classmate's cruel comment about her weight speaks to her insecurities, serving as a catalyst for the onset of her eating disorder. The book details the 53 days that Riley receives treatment for anorexia nervosa at an eating disorder treatment facility. Riley documents her experience in treatment through private journal entries. Throughout her entries, Riley shares how the voice in her head, named "Ed" (an acronym for *eating disorder*), tells her she isn't good enough—not as a daughter, not as a sister, not as a friend, not as a runner, not as an artist. Riley recounts her sessions with her therapist, Willow, and her experiences getting to know the other patients and forging new friendships. Riley's interactions with her family, her friends, and the other patients illustrate the pressures that many adolescents face. As the book progresses, Riley learns to recognize her own strength and to self-advocate in her journey toward seeing herself as "good enough," de-emphasizing perfection and focusing on embracing all aspects of being human.

GUIDING STUDENTS INTO THE TEXT

Mental Health Literacy

Petro-Roy offers a realistic portrayal of adolescent eating disorder treatment in her novel. The author shares concepts in her book that are unique to the culture of eating disorder treatment that will be useful to understand as an educator who is preparing to engage students in the reading of this novel. Terms in the following list that do not indicate day numbers for journal entries are those concepts woven frequently throughout the book.

- *Eating disorders:* Describes a complex biopsychosocial disease that manifests as a product of genetics, temperament, environmental factors, and stress and concerns an unhealthy obsession with food, weight, and body image (Wood & Schneider, 2015).
- *Anorexia nervosa:* A type of eating disorder that is characterized by restriction of food intake, low body weight, an intense fear of gaining weight, and a disturbance of how one experiences their body (APA, 2013).
- *Bulimia nervosa:* A type of eating disorder characterized by cycles of binge eating followed by behaviors of purging, such as self-induced vomiting, to undo the effects and feelings associated with binging (APA, 2013).
- *Binge eating disorder:* A type of eating disorder characterized by repeatedly eating large quantities of food and experiencing feelings during the binge episode, for example, shame, loss of control, or guilt, and not using purge behaviors afterward (APA, 2013).
- *Shame:* An intense negative feeling characterized by the perception that one is defective or worthless in some way (Tangney & Dearing, 2002).
- *Observations (OBS):* A treatment protocol used in many eating disorder facilities to support clients in stopping eating disorder behaviors, for example, purging or exercising, in high-risk situations such as using the bathroom after meals (Day 2).
- *Eating disorder urge:* The rising feeling in one's body felt before engaging in an eating disorder behavior such as restricting, binging, purging, or overexercising (Fitzsimmons-Craft et al., 2016).

Initially, clients may not be in touch with their behavioral urges. Successful treatment includes clients coming into awareness with these urges and learning to connect urges to feelings and manage the feelings with a healthier coping strategy (Day 42).

- *Perfectionism:* A mindset that rejects and fears failure and/or constructive feedback, with an all-or-nothing approach (Ben-Shahar, 2009).
- *Fat-phobia:* A pathological fear and stigmatization of fatness (Day 9) (Bacon et al., 2001).

English Language Arts Literacy

Before beginning to read the book, teachers can introduce students to the five main narrator points of view: first person, second person, third-person objective, third-person limited, and third-person omniscient. Teachers can provide a selection of books for students to browse in pairs to determine the author's point of view (see table 3.1 for a sample of texts). Students can work together to identify the point of view, provide evidence for their thinking, and share with the class in a whole-class discussion. The objective for introducing point of view is to form the basis of deeper analysis of why an author develops a specific point of view for the narrator in a text so that students might later engage in critical analysis of character development and perspective taking within the story. As students engage in their reading of *Good Enough*, they will revisit point of view and use this foundational understanding to develop

Table 3.1. Introduction to Point of View (POV): A Sampling of Texts

Title	Author	POV	Evidence
Almost Paradise	Corabel Shofner	first person	Use of "I"
Bud, Not Buddy	Christopher Paul Curtis	first person	Use of "I"
Roll of Thunder, Hear My Cry	Mildred D. Taylor	first person	Use of "I"
Moon Mission: The Epic 400-Year Journey to Apollo 11	Sigmund Brouwer	second person	Use of "You"
You Can Fly: The Tuskegee Airmen	Carole Boston Weatherford	second person	Use of "You"
Blackbird	Anna Carey	second person	Use of "You"
Hoot	Carl Hiaasen	third person	Use of "He"
Touching Spirit Bear	Ben Mikaelsen	third person	Use of "He"
Tuck Everlasting	Natalie Babbitt	third person	Use of "She"

their critical interpretations of the text, character development, and the narrator's vantage point related to the events within the story.

Exploring the Author's Note

Petro-Roy reveals to the reader that, like Riley, she was also diagnosed with anorexia nervosa, along with exercise addiction. She shares that she suffered from issues with food and self-esteem for years before her eating disorder came to light. More important, she alludes to the fact that her feelings of inadequacy are not the reason for her eating disorder. Rather, in addition to a complex biopsychosocial genetic makeup, her eating disorder gave her an identity, which in return allowed her to feel special. Through treatment and therapy, she learned that she is good enough; that having an eating disorder does not make her special, but embracing her humanness and being herself does. Pre-reading the author's note with students will help them understand what anorexia nervosa is and is not. It is a manifestation of many different things and, most important, not an attention-seeking behavior.

You Are Enough: Your Guide to Body Image and Eating Disorder Recovery, also by Petro-Roy, is a nonfiction self-help companion to *Good Enough* that brings readers on the author's journey to recovery. It is an inclusive guide that discusses eating disorders and body image; it also provides information on available treatments and relaxation techniques. The author also included the websites for the National Eating Disorders Association (https://www.nationaleatingdisorders.org/help-support) and National Association of Anorexia Nervosa and Associated Disorders (https://anad.org/get-help). Additionally, as previously mentioned, the Health at Every Size Model also provides clear guidelines that can support further discussion and resources (https://haescommunity.com).

Introducing and Practicing Metaphor and Simile

Throughout *Good Enough*, Petro-Roy provides readers a glimpse into Riley's experience, connections with characters, and character development through the ongoing use of metaphors and similes. Riley's journal entries are filled with figurative language that depicts her views of fellow patients, family members, and her inner emotions, along with reflections on her experience in treatment. Additionally, the use of metaphor in the treatment of eating disorders is also quite effective in that it allows individuals to discuss difficult topics in a more manageable way. Before reading the novel, teachers can introduce students to the structure and purpose of similes and metaphors so that readers are able to later identify and critically analyze this figurative language found throughout the text.

As so many of Riley's similes and metaphors demonstrate her evolving considerations and feelings toward her eating disorder, as well as her perceptions of others, it can be helpful for students to begin by creating collaborative and personal examples to represent some of their own experiences and perceptions of themes found throughout the novel. After introducing students to definitions for simile and metaphor, teachers can collaborate with students to construct unique metaphors and similes that represent student understanding of themes such as friendship, family, identity, self-discovery, personal growth, change, and "normal." For example, the class might work together to construct metaphors and similes that speak to their communal understanding of friendship, as well as those that speak to their unique views and experiences with friendship (see table 3.2). The class can then examine how their similes and metaphors are similar or different from one another, as well as how each metaphor and simile speaks to their unique perspective. In the same way that the therapists in the book do not talk about each other's bodies, due to the competitive nature of eating disorders, educators should avoid having students use metaphor to describe bodies in the event students have undisclosed struggles with food.

Finally, teachers can engage students in conversation surrounding how their unique views of each key theme speak to their individual perspective, experience, and identity. As they prepare to read *Good Enough*, students can consider how Riley's use of metaphor and simile will represent her unique perspective and journey throughout the pages of the novel.

Table 3.2. Practice with Simile and Metaphor Example

Topic Selection	Class Simile	My Simile	Class Metaphor	My Metaphor	Significance to My Perspective
Friendship	Friendship is like a roller coaster. Ups and downs. Twists and turns.	Friendship is like a delicate flower. It requires care and attention if it is going to bloom.	Friendship is a bracelet. Each person contributes a strand—weaving together to create something beautiful.	Friendship is a summer day. Beautiful. Fun. Full of possibility. Watch for the afternoon storms.	My perspective is unique because my friendships are few, unique, and special to me.
Family	Family is like a solid oak tree. We have our roots, but we also have our branches. We grow where we are planted.	Family is like a tree with deep roots and wide branches.	Family is a security blanket. Always there if you find yourself in need of care and comfort.	Family is a patchwork quilt. We all come from the same cloth, but we are each unique in our own way.	My perspective is unique because my family is important to me. I would do anything for my family.

GUIDING STUDENTS THROUGH THE TEXT

Tracking Character Development

Character development is linked to point of view. In a book written in first-person perspective, the reader will have a strong sense of the protagonist but may have a limited understanding of secondary characters. This is because the story is being told from the main character's point of view. To help students understand this, teachers can have readers track the development of the protagonist, along with a selection of secondary characters, throughout the book. Students can examine their evolving impressions of the characters, their impressions and understanding of the lead protagonist, and the impact of secondary characters on the story. For the purpose of *Good Enough*, students might choose to focus on characters such as Riley, Julia, Riley's mom, Ali, Willow, and Brenna. For the purpose of the example chart provided here (table 3.3), we have given attention to Riley and Julia's characters. As the characters are introduced in the novel, teachers can prompt students to think about what they know about the character with such guiding questions as the following:

- What information about the character has Riley shared in her journal?
- What is your initial impression as a result of this information?
- What more would you like to know about this character?
- In what ways might Riley's perspective of this character be biased? And why is this significant to consider?
- When might "Ed" be the one journaling versus Riley's true self?

Students will repeat this activity as they continue their reading of the book and at the conclusion of the novel so they can think about how their impressions and understandings of the character might have changed or developed throughout the course of the novel. Students can also consider how Riley's interpretation of each secondary character speaks to the reader's developing impressions and understanding of Riley's persona.

Table 3.3. Character Development Chart Partial Example

Character	First Impressions (Beginning)	Getting to Know You (During)	Lasting Impressions (End)	In What Ways Did This Character Change?	Why Do You Think This Character Changed? (Catalyst for Change)
Riley	It seems like Riley is misunderstood. She thinks she's not that sick, but everyone thinks she is.	Riley thinks she knows what other people think about her but isn't always right.	Riley was good at hiding her feelings, and this contributed to her eating disorder.	Riley changed by being willing to talk about her problems, learned to express her feelings, and let others help her.	I think Riley changed because she had help from Willow and because she wanted to get better and took a risk to share her feelings.
Julia	It seems Julia is dedicated to gymnastics. She is worried about her older sister.	Julia really cares about her sister. During her visits, you can tell Julia has a strong bond with Riley and wants her sister to feel better.	Julia is a thoughtful, considerate character who seems to listen and love others for who they are on the inside.	I don't know if Julia changed throughout the story except that in the beginning she was noted to be sad and worried, and by the end, she seems happy and eager to be with Riley again.	I think the catalyst for change for Julia was her ability to listen and think of others.

At the conclusion of the novel, readers might come to see that not only do they know a great deal more about the main character but also what they have come to know about the others is based on the protagonist's perspective.

Perspectives on Moments in Time

In addition to tracking readers' impressions of characters, teachers can encourage students to think more deeply about character development and its relationship to point of view through the consideration of character response to key moments in the story. Students can consider what they know about the main character and a supporting character of their choice as they examine how each character might perceive and respond to a particular event from the text. For example, teachers might select key moments in the plot of the story, such as the "Ed Group" gatherings (p. 76), the group's goodbye party for Brenna (p. 182), or the family meeting between Riley and her mom, dad, and counselor (p. 191), which feature multiple characters from the novel. Students can pause to consider how each of the characters involved in the experience act or respond to the conflict or moment at hand. They can then consider how the experience is filtered through Riley's perspective, and the impact of this single perspective on the reader's growing understanding and interpretation of each character. Students can maintain ongoing reading journals to accompany their character development charts (see table 3.3). As they approach the conclusion of the novel, students can draw upon their collection of notes and information to further their character analysis and conclusions. Teachers can jumpstart student reflection by providing journal prompts such as the following:

- How does the character respond in this situation?
- How does the character feel in this situation? What has led you to this conclusion?
- How might Riley's perspective of this moment in time impact the reader's perception of the character?
- Is there another way to view this situation?
- How might the character perceive this moment in time if the story were told from his/her/their perspective?

As they compose their reading journals, students should note the page number, provide a brief description of the key event or conflict taking place in the story, and then consider each of the provided journal prompts as they continue in their character analysis.

Tracking Character Development through Simile and Metaphor

Another essential means of tracking character development throughout *Good Enough* is through critical examination of metaphors and similes as they are interspersed throughout Riley's journal entries. Riley draws upon a wide range of metaphors and similes as she documents her experience in treatment. Readers can note how Riley's evolving views of her family, fellow patients, and Ed contribute to her character development and journey toward recovery. As her days in treatment progress, students can take note of how the metaphors and similes not only reveal more about the secondary characters as shared through Riley's unique perspective but also how changes in Riley's selection of such figurative language demonstrate essential shifts in her perspective of her eating disorder recovery and personal goals in progressing through treatment. For example, on Day 1, Riley refers to the treatment facility as "solitary confinement. Like we're lab animals shut up in a box and part of some big experiment" (p. 9). By Day 29, Riley writes, "It felt like someone had let me out of a jail cell after I'd been sentenced to life in prison, except instead of my body, it was my brain that was free" (p. 212). Teachers can use a graphic organizer similar to the example provided in table 3.4 to assist students in tracking the use of similes and metaphors, the meaning readers associate with each example, and how the noted examples speak to Riley's character and development throughout the course of the novel.

As students near the conclusion of the novel, teachers can also revisit students' initial metaphors and similes (see table 3.2) and work together to identify how Riley's use of metaphor and simile speak to her own views of the previously identified themes and how those views might have changed or developed throughout the course of the novel. As students engage in critical examination of Riley's metaphors and similes, they can gain additional insight into the role of perspective and character development through figurative language.

Table 3.4. Riley's Journey through Metaphor and Simile Example

Day in Treatment	Passage from the Text	Simile or Metaphor	What Does This Mean?	What Might This Reveal about Riley?
Day 1	"She had one hand on my shoulder, her fingernails as sharp as an eagle's talons. I was the mouse, wriggling to get free."	Simile (eagle talons and nails); metaphor (I was the mouse)	Riley is describing her mom's grip on her arm the day her parents were taking her to the treatment facility.	Riley feels trapped by her mother. She doesn't think anything is wrong with her and feels that her mother is forcing her to go.
Day 1	"This whole place feels like solitary confinement. Like we're lab animals shut up in a box and part of some big experiment."	Simile (lab animals and the patients)	Riley feels like she and the other patients are all being watched and trapped in treatment.	Riley perceives treatment as something she is being forced to do. She feels like others are watching her, testing her, and experimenting on her like she were nothing more than a lab rat.
Day 2	"I had to turn my attention back to my food mountain then, the one I have to climb six times a day. Each step I take, it gets steeper and steeper."	Metaphor (food and a mountain)	Riley is describing her views of the meals she eats while in treatment.	Riley seems to perceive this aspect of treatment as challenging—like climbing a mountain.

Combining HAES and Point of View

There are moments in the text when Riley writes from the point of view of her eating disorder. For example, on Day 9, Riley documents a dialogue between her Healthy Voice and Ed as the two argue over Riley's decision to reveal her true feelings to her therapist, Willow (p. 107). On Day 15, Riley's Healthy Voice and Ed debate her decision to engage in exercise against the expectations of treatment (p. 140).

Teachers can have students take note of this internal struggle, not only to expand upon their understanding of point of view but also to practice the HAES concepts of compassionate self-care and respect for all bodies. Compassionate self-care encourages attunement with ourselves—not only how we move and eat in the world but also how we treat and honor our bodies and the bodies of others. In this exercise, students can select a part of the body of a character in the novel and write from the point of view of that body part using a compassionate lens (see table 3.5). Students can think about how the selected body part helps the character in the book, despite its size or aesthetic appearance. Teachers can use the prompt: "If (name of character) (part of body) could speak, what would it say?"

After the exercise, students can reflect on what it was like to write from the point of view of a body part. They might consider: What did they learn about point of view through the activity? What did the activity

Table 3.5.   Example HAES and POV Chart

Character	Part of Body	From a HAES Perspective, What a Character's Body Part Might Say	Location in Book
Riley	Eyes	I am Riley's eyes. I help Riley by looking at the subjects she draws for her art pieces and work together with her hand to help her make art. I love to watch movies.	Day 22
Brenna	Hands	I am Brenna's hands, and I am awesome! I can make cool comics and do puzzles with Riley!	Day 9
Ali	Abdominals	I am Ali's abdominals. She makes me do crunches every night. I am exhausted. I wish I could just relax and be me.	Day 4
Willow	Mouth	I am Willow's mouth. I help speak truths to my clients to support them. I know how to set boundaries with clients. I make clients feel comfortable with my warm smile.	Day 3

reveal about their understanding of the character or their perspective of the character? How did such an activity speak to their understanding of the HAES model?

Discussion Questions

As teachers work through the book, there are many rich areas to engage students. In the following list, we have highlighted some key areas, starting with specific pages to discuss and then ending with more broad discussion questions after completing the text.

- On Day 1, Riley says, "Potential is what everyone has. Everyone but me. I'm the boring one" (p. 6). Why do you think she says this? Do you believe it is possible for everyone to have potential except one person in the world?
- The technique of personification is used in treatment and in literature. In the novel, the eating disorder is personified as Ed. On Day 4, Riley says, "Ed might be a liar, but he makes me feel better. He makes me forget about everything else that's going on. He makes me believe, if only for a little while, that my body will be okay, even if everything else might not be" (p. 81). One way to think of an eating disorder, disordered eating, or obsession with how we look is to think of it like a misguided hero that is trying to protect someone the best way they know how. In what other ways do you see how Riley's eating disorder has protected her? What does Riley have to learn to do in treatment to protect and care for herself in more healthy ways?
- On Day 5, Riley discusses talking with others in group therapy, noting, "It surprises me every time someone in here thinks like me. I am so used to feeling like 'the only one'" (p. 84). Why do you think talking about things that are hard to discuss is helpful for Riley and others in treatment?
- On Day 9, Riley's friend in treatment, Brenna, talks about being fat. The therapist says, "You're right, Brenna. . . . What's so bad about being fat?" Riley ponders this, asking the following questions: "Does being skinny make you a better person?" "Does eating

less food make you more kind?" "Is eating too much food a crime?" (pp. 108–9). How would you respond? Support students in referring to the HAES Model if they get stuck in their own biases.

- Discuss times in the book where Riley made assumptions about other characters' thinking. Why do you think people make assumptions? How do assumptions act as a protective function? Is it possible that they can hurt people?
- Respect and compassion toward oneself and others is part of what allows Riley to accept being in her body. Discuss times in the book where Riley learned to respect her body or respected the body of another character. Who helps her learn to do this? Why is respecting bodies of all shapes and sizes important?
- When Riley goes on her pass, she has success at dinner with her friends but struggles at breakfast with her family (pp. 230–41). What do you think allowed Riley to be successful at dinner? Why do you think she struggled at breakfast?
- In what ways do you think journaling or creating art helps Riley? Why do you think the author chose to write this story using the first-person point of view?
- At the end of the book, Riley gets to put her snowflake up and let go of her fears (p. 261). What surprised you about her fears?

GUIDING STUDENTS OUT OF THE TEXT

A Call to Action

This section integrates meaningful activities that allow teachers and students to take the mental health aspects of the novel and apply them to their school settings in service of concretizing what they learned and transitioning out from the novel.

The Masks We Wear

We all have ways that we protect ourselves. For Riley, the mask of the eating disorder is what protects her. Carl Rogers (1995) coined the term *incongruent*, which is when we feel one way on the inside but show the world another way on the outside. That feeling of being incongruent is often what leaves people feeling inauthentic or less happy. For Riley, she had to learn to stop letting the eating disorder protect her by pushing down her emotions but, rather, share those emotions with others. When her inside and outside matched, and she witnessed that her world did not crumble, she stopped feeling inauthentic and started to feel good enough. One way that Riley explored herself was through journaling and through her art.

First, teachers can have students identify some of the feelings Riley felt on the inside that were hard to share or show on the outside. Teachers can ask students to discuss how Riley learned to have compassion for herself through her journey and provide students a paper outline of a mask (see figure 3.1). Using colors, words, or collage images from magazines, students can represent what Riley showed to the world on the front side of the mask; students can then represent feelings or parts that Riley felt she could not show to the world on the back of the mask (i.e., inside). Students can make use of words, along with images and colors, to express Riley's feelings. Afterward, teachers may invite students to share their work with a partner, exploring similarities and differences that the students portrayed from their viewpoints.

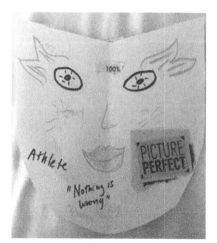 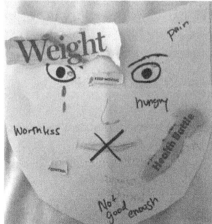

Figure 3.1. Example Front (Left) and Back (Right) of Mask

HAES in the School Setting

Riley came to understand how important her body was, and how all bodies are worthwhile of being nourished, receiving care and compassion, and being respected. Riley points out in her journal a great example of how products are marketed in American society that are focused on thinness and sexualizing individuals: "There is an entire section on the menu called 'Skinnylicious,' which is pretty much the dumbest thing ever. I don't want to be anything-licious. It's all diet food and there are calories listed next to each option and I'm pretty much freaking out" (p. 231). In this exercise, students can work to make their school environment a more socially just and accepting place that honors every body's inherent worth, no matter what size. Using the HAES principles of respect and compassionate care, teachers can put students into small groups and ask them to brainstorm messages that would convey that every student's body in the school is a worthwhile one, or messages about students' worth beyond the size of their body. Student groups can share out and select a few favorite statements from those shared with the class. Students can then write down these selected sentiments on brightly colored sticky notes. Teachers can provide each student with five sticky notes to take with them at the end of class and invite them to place sticky notes on students' lockers, bathroom mirrors, or other places that would help create a more positive and affirming environment.

Closing the Book

Reimagining the Scene

As a way to assess that students understand the role that point of view has in character development, teachers can invite them to rewrite a scene in the book from another character's perspective in the form of a secondary character's journal entry. Students might choose from the following: Julia (Day 1), Ali (Day 4), Riley's mom (Day 18), Brenna (Day 30), or Emerson or Josie (Day 41). Students should be sure to add internal thoughts for these characters that do not exist in *Good Enough* because of the first-person point of view. For example, the journal entry featured in figure 3.2 represents Julia's experience on Day 1 as Riley enters treatment.

Day 1 without Riley

Riley hasn't been away long, and I already miss her so much! How could Mom and Dad spring this on me last night?!?! How could they hide this from me for so long?!

How could *Riley* keep this from me? I mean, did she even know? Or, did Mom and Dad just throw this at her, too??

I know she needs this. I have noticed changes for a while now. I've been worried about her, but I didn't want to say anything. I worried if I said something... it would be true – that something was wrong. I know I am busy. It's hard to keep up with school, my friends, and gymnastics. Is it my fault that Riley had to go away today? Could I have been a better sister? Should I have said something to mom and dad? Did keeping all of this a secret hurt her?

I can't stop crying! This just stinks!!! I miss my sister!! The house feels so small – so empty when she's not right across the hallway.

Mom and Dad keep trying to act like things are okay, but we all know they're not. No one spoke much today. Mom was on the phone most of the day trying to figure out stuff at the Gallery. Dad kept to himself (no surprise there). I couldn't focus on my routine and almost fell on my face at practice.

I told her "Good luck" as she headed out. I had to keep things together for her. But, now I'm just falling   apart... I hope she comes home soon! Please, Riley... Come home soon. I can't do this without you.

Figure 3.2. Julia's Journal Entry

CONCLUSION

Petro-Roy makes clear that she is in her own eating disorder recovery and is a passionate advocate for eating disorder awareness. By using *Good Enough* as a text in the classroom, students are exposed to the seriousness of eating disorders and the feelings that underlie them. The text, in conjunction with the strategies outlined in this chapter, will allow students to gain a deeper understanding of ways that people protect themselves with an eating disorder. Additionally, students will hopefully feel encouraged to compassionately honor their unique bodies and qualities of themselves and their peers, while understanding the impact of the author's choice of using point-of-view narrative as a literary style for the novel.

REFERENCES

American Psychiatric Association. (2013). *Diagnostic and statistical manual of mental disorders* (5th ed.). Washington, DC: American Psychiatric Publishing. https://doi.org/10.1176/appi.books.9780890425596

Bacon, J. G., Scheltema, K. E., & Robinson, B. E. (2001). Fat phobia scale revisited: The short form. *International Journal of Obesity*, 25(2), 252–57. https://doi.org/10.1038/sj.ijo.0801537

Bacon, L. (2010). *Health at every size: The surprising truth about your weight.* Dallas, TX: BenBella Books.

Ben-Shahar, T. (2009). *The pursuit of perfect.* Prince Frederick, MD: High-Bridge.

Bucchianeri, M. M., Arikian, A. J., Hannan, P. J., Eisenberg, M. E., & Neumark-Sztainer, D. (2013). Body dissatisfaction from adolescence to young adulthood: Findings from a 10-year longitudinal study. *Body Image*, 10(1). https://doi.org/10.1016/j.bodyim.2012.09.001

Cass, K., McGuire, C., Bjork, I., Sobotka, N., Walsh, K., & Mehler, P. S. (2020). Medical complications of anorexia nervosa. *Psychosomatics*, 61(6), 625–31. https://doi.org/10.1016/j.psym.2020.06.020

Clare, M. M., Ardron-Hudson, E. A., & Grindell, J. (2015). Fat in school: Applied interdisciplinarity as a basis for consultation in oppressive social context. *Journal of Educational and Psychological Consultation*, 25(1), 45–65. https://doi.org/10.1080/10474412.2014.929952

Fitzsimmons-Craft, E. E., Ciao, A. C., & Accurso, E. C. (2016). A naturalistic examination of social comparisons and disordered eating thoughts, urges, and behaviors in college women. *International Journal of Eating Disorders*, 49(2), 141–50. https://doi.org/10.1002/eat.22486

Kater, K. (2012). *Healthy bodies: Teaching kids what they need to know.* North St. Paul, MN: Body Image Health.

Marengo, D., Longobardi, C., Fabris, M. A., & Settanni, M. (2018). Highly-visual social media and internalizing symptoms in adolescence: The mediating role of body image concerns. *Computers in Human Behavior*, 82, 63–69. https://doi.org/10.1016/j.chb.2018.01.003

Mills, J. S., Shannon, A., & Hogue, J. (2017). Beauty, body image, and the media. In *Perception of beauty* (pp. 145–57). IntechOpen. https://doi.org/10.5772/intechopen.68944

Murray, S. B., Pila, E., Griffiths, S., & Le Grange, D. (2017). When illness severity and research dollars do not align: Are we overlooking eating disorders? *World Psychiatry*, 16(3), 321. https://doi.og/10.1002/wps.20465

Petro-Roy, J. (2019). *Good enough.* New York: Square Fish.

Pike, K. M., & Rodin, J. (1991). Mothers, daughters, and disordered eating. *Journal of Abnormal Psychology*, 100(2), 198–204. https://doi.org/10.1037//0021-843x.100.2.198

Ridder, M. (2020). Revenue of the beauty and cosmetic industry in the United States from 2002 to 2020. *Statista*. https://www.statista.com/statistics/243742/revenue-of-the-cosmetic-industry-in-the-us/

Rogers, C. R. (1995). *On becoming a person: A therapist's view of psychotherapy*. Boston, MA: Houghton Mifflin Harcourt.

Saunders, J. F., & Eaton, A. A. (2018). Snaps, selfies, and shares: How three popular social media platforms contribute to the sociocultural model of disordered eating among young women. *Cyberpsychology, Behavior, and Social Networking, 21*(6), 343–54. https://doi.org/10.1089/cyber.2017.0713

Schwartz, R. C., & Sweezy, M. (2019). *Internal family systems therapy*. New York: Guilford.

Tangney, J. P., & Dearing, R. L. (2002). *Shame and guilt*. New York: Guilford.

Wood, L. L. (2015). Eating disorder as protector: The use of internal family systems and drama therapy to help clients understand the protective function of their eating disorders. In A. Heidescheit (Ed.), *Creative arts therapies and clients with eating disorders* (pp. 293–325). Philadelphia, PA: Jessica Kingsley.

Wood, L. L., & Schneider, C. (2015). Setting the stage for self-attunement: Drama therapy as a guide for neural integration in the treatment of eating disorders. *Drama Therapy Review, 1*(1), 55–70. https://doi.org/10.1386/dtr.1.1.55_1

4

SECRECY, SILENCE, AND TRANSGENERATIONAL TRAUMA

Conflict and Character Development in
I Am Not Your Perfect Mexican Daughter

Daniela Bustamante and Katie Sciurba

Trauma and hardship of any kind are difficult issues to discuss. In an effort to avoid feelings of shame, guilt, sadness, or distress that may arise when talking about trauma, many people will keep difficult personal experiences a secret. Teens in particular may avoid discussing trauma as they attempt to fit into behavioral and experiential norms they observe among their peers (Telzer et al., 2018). While the desire to fit in is natural, a culture of secrecy in response to hardships can prevent access to support and care during a time where teens may be more susceptible to mental health concerns and risks, such as depression or risky behavior. In 2017, the Centers for Disease Control (CDC) reported a 28 percent increase in suicide rates in the past 15 years and noted that suicide was the third leading cause of death for children between the ages of 10 and 14, and the second leading cause of death for young people between 15 and 24 (Stone et al., 2017). Evidence shows that second-generation teens (i.e., the generation first born in a country after their parents immigrated from another place) show higher rates of depression and substance use, and they are nearly three times as likely to attempt suicide as their peers (Peña et al., 2008). Children of immigrant parents are also at an increased risk for experiencing transgenerational trauma, as immigrants and refugees often experience severe hardship or trauma prior to, during, and after immigrating to a new country (Phipps & Degges-White, 2014).

As Dutro (2019) discusses, the "hard stuff of life" is inevitably present in every classroom, experienced by students and teachers alike (p. 1). Using literature and narratives as tools for exploration allows students to give "shape and meaning to the worlds we inhabit" and to recognize and process their own experiences through the safe containers of characters and stories (Dutro, 2019, p. 78). Along with naming and unpacking mental health and cultural influences through exploring fictional texts, educators can deepen students' understandings of character development (how a character transforms as a story unfolds). For instance, adolescent readers can explore how the personal hardships of protagonists and their families shape who they are and how they relate to one another, as well as how their senses of self and their relationships evolve. Adolescent readers can also identify sources of conflict (the struggle between two opposing forces) present in a story, while acknowledging the distinction between external and internal conflict. In addition to discussing the conflict *between* characters, it is just as valuable to explore the conflicts characters face within themselves.

The young adult novel *I Am Not Your Perfect Mexican Daughter* by Erika L. Sánchez (2017) explores how secrecy in response to trauma can have negative effects for many people, not just the secret-keeper. Sánchez explores how stressful events can affect a family across generations, and how secrecy leads to conflict, misunderstandings, and more serious consequences for many characters. Exploring the effects of trauma and secrecy on the characters in the story, *I Am Not Your Perfect Mexican Daughter* can teach readers to recognize the consequences of remaining silent while struggling internally, to explore various coping strategies to manage personal distress, and to develop empathy for people with diverse identities and backgrounds. Through activities addressing character conflicts and Julia's journey toward self-acceptance, students can gain understandings of character complexity and story development.

UNDERSTANDING TRANSGENERATIONAL TRAUMA

Many people may be familiar with the idea of trauma as experiencing a stressful or upsetting event that causes lasting effects on a person's behavior and emotional well-being. In the case of transgenerational trauma, the effects of the traumatic event are not direct but, rather, are transmitted from the original victims to subsequent generations. As an individual's behavior, attitudes, and beliefs about the world are influenced by their personal trauma, it shapes their interactions with loved ones and family members, including their children and grandchildren (Phipps & Degges-White, 2014). This in turn allows the effects of the original trauma to influence the beliefs, attitudes, and behavior of subsequent generations, leading to a transgenerational legacy. Transgenerational trauma can have individual familial effects, or it can be more widespread, such as in the case of wars, famines, plagues, or other large-scale events affecting groups of people. Because of tendencies toward secrecy and silence in response to personal trauma, it is often the case that individuals may not tell their family about their experiences. This can make effects of transgenerational trauma harder to recognize or acknowledge, as subsequent generations might be entirely unaware of the original trauma despite its lasting influence (Phipps & Degges-White, 2014).

I AM NOT YOUR PERFECT MEXICAN DAUGHTER BY ERIKA L. SÁNCHEZ

Fifteen-year-old Julia is the younger daughter of Mexican immigrants living in Chicago with her parents and older sister, Olga. The story opens with the death of Olga, who was—in everyone's view—the perfect Mexican daughter. Julia's parents are devastated over the loss of their perfect child, who cooked and cleaned, spoke only Spanish at home, never went out at night, and chose to live at home to stay with her family after high school. Julia is nothing like Olga—she dreams of leaving home to attend college in New York City, wants to go out with her friends and new boyfriend Connor, and has no interest in learning how to make tortillas or having a traditional *quinceañera* to celebrate her coming of age.

In addition to managing the everyday stresses of being a teenager, Julia must deal with her own grief at the loss of her sister, her parents' grief, and the pressures and expectations placed on her as the surviving daughter and as a second-generation Mexican American stuck between her parents' native culture and her own. Julia begins to learn secrets about her sister, her parents, and her friends, and she keeps secrets about herself, as well. As she uncovers and begins to grapple with these secrets, Julia gains a deeper understanding of the people around her and a stronger sense of who she is and what it means to live her life on her own terms.

GUIDING STUDENTS INTO THE TEXT

Mental Health Literacy

The book is narrated from the first-person perspective of a teenager who is not well acquainted with mental health issues. As such, the text does not use specific mental health terminology or clearly identify each instance where a character is struggling with mental health concerns. Instead, the text provides descriptions of the behaviors of individuals who are experiencing these states, such as the way Julia describes her mother in the weeks following Olga's death: staying in bed, not showering or getting dressed, and barely eating or drinking. After Olga's funeral, Julia also notices that Amá cannot take care of her typical responsibilities, such as grocery shopping, cleaning the house, or working (chapter 2). Although it is never explicitly stated, these observations illustrate symptoms that, when occurring together, indicate the likelihood of depression: a decrease in appetite, sleeping excessively and feeling fatigued, loss of interest in typical activities, and impairment in normal social and professional function (American Psychiatric Association [APA], 2013).

The following concept definitions can help unfamiliar readers recognize and categorize the behaviors that are described throughout the book (some of these terms have been defined in other chapters of this text, and can be referred to for additional detail):

- *Trauma:* A response to a highly stressful life event or events, such as exposure to death, injury, or sexual, physical, or emotional violence. Trauma causes an individual to experience a heightened sense of risk and lack of safety—even after the stressful event is no longer happening—and can affect a person's ability to cope health-ily with stress moving forward (Trauma and Learning Policy Initia-tive, 2013). Possible responses to trauma can include depression, anxiety, physical "flashbacks" to the stressful event, and feeling unsafe in personal relationships.

- *Posttraumatic stress disorder (PTSD):* A psychiatric diagnosis given to people who show a particular cluster of multiple responses to trauma that are severe enough to affect a person's ability to func-tion at work or school, to form healthy relationships, and to feel satisfied in their daily life. It is important to note that not every individual who experiences trauma develops PTSD, and this diag-nosis can only be determined by a health professional (APA, 2013).
- *Depression:* An emotional state where a person has a consistently down or sad mood and experiences changes to their typical daily activities. Some people experience depression without a noted cause, but it can also occur in response to a specific experience, such as trauma. Depression can include loss of interest or enjoy-ment in activities that were once enjoyable, changes in weight or appetite, changes in sleep pattern, loss of energy, physical agitation, irritability, feelings of worthlessness or guilt, difficulty focusing and making decisions, and thoughts of death or self-harm (Centers for Disease Control [CDC], 2020).
- *Anxiety:* A state of fear or worry that can disrupt a person's ability to function or participate in their typical activities. Anxiety can cause obsessive and intrusive thoughts that affect focus and sleep, agita-tion or irritability, and physical symptoms such as upset stomach, difficulty breathing, racing heart, or feeling jittery (CDC, 2020).
- *Grief:* A response to significant loss, such as a death, one's home, or other disruptions to personal relationships. Expressions of grief can vary depending on cultural norms but can involve symptoms simi-lar to depression. Unlike typical depression, grief only occurs in the context of a loss (or an anticipated loss) and typically becomes less intense over time (Corless et al., 2014).
- *Suicide:* An intentional act meant to end one's own life or kill one-self, often related to episodes of depression and hopelessness (Peña et al., 2008).

- *Survivor's guilt:* A symptom in which a survivor of a traumatic event feels guilty or undeserving of surviving an incident that could have caused them more serious harm or death, where others were harmed or killed (APA, 2013).

"What Is Trauma?" Jigsaw Activity

Prior to beginning the book study, students can work together to examine the broad concept of trauma and learn about its various manifestations through a jigsaw activity. Dividing the class into small groups, teachers can assign students to explore research questions connected to the trauma-related terms described in the previous section. Possible research questions to explore include the following:

1. What causes trauma?
2. What are possible symptoms of trauma and PTSD?
3. What causes transgenerational trauma?
4. What is the difference between grief and depression?
5. What are symptoms of depression?
6. What are symptoms of anxiety?
7. What professional supports are available for people who experience trauma?

Students can consult various primary and secondary sources to gather data related to their research questions. The jigsaw project is an opportunity for educators to partner with resources within the school and local communities, and for students to learn research and inquiry skills. School media specialists can guide students in conducting independent research and determining credible sources in both print and online settings. Furthermore, school mental health professionals can be consulted for resources about trauma and can give information about in-school services and supports available for coping with trauma. Community partnerships can include invited speakers or interviews with Public Health Department officials, local university or college professors working in mental health or counseling-related departments, as well as local mental health care professionals.

Each student group can gather three substantial findings (or answers) in response to their research questions to present to the rest of the class,

Term Explored (e.g. "Trauma")	
Research Questions: What causes trauma? What are some symptoms of trauma and PTSD?	Sources Consulted: 1. *Psychological Trauma*: Book by Bessel A. van der Kolk 2. *Children and Trauma*: Pamphlet published by the International Society for Traumatic Stress Studies (ISTSS) 3. *What Is Complex Trauma: A Resource Guide for Youth and Those Who Care about Them*: Pamphlet published by the National Child Trauma Stress Network (NCTSN)
Findings: 1. Trauma is caused by experiencing an upsetting and stressful event or events. Examples of upsetting events include car accidents, natural disasters, war, sexual assault, physical or emotional abuse, or death. A person can experience more than one traumatic event in their life, which can cause more serious trauma reactions. 2. A traumatized person is affected even after the traumatic experience is over, and they might feel unsafe all the time or fear that something else bad is going to happen to them. In some cases, the person can be diagnosed with a disorder called posttraumatic stress disorder (PTSD). 3. Trauma symptoms can include feeling depressed or sad, scared or anxious that other bad things will happen, and feeling unsafe even when nothing bad is happening. Sometimes people might have nightmares or imagine that the traumatic event is happening to them again, or they might react to other upsetting experiences because it reminds them of their trauma. In PTSD, people experience many trauma symptoms instead of just a few.	

Figure 4.1. "What Is Trauma?" Sample Poster

either as a series of multimedia presentations or poster of the findings (see figure 4.1 for a sample poster template).

Coping Skills

Coping skills are activities and behaviors that can be used to help a person deal with or "cope" with their emotions and experiences. Coping skills can take many different forms that serve different purposes in helping someone feel better. Not every person will benefit from every coping skill, and preferences will vary; however, "coping flexibility"— that is, being able to access and use a wider variety of coping skills—has been associated with better emotional adjustment and lower rates of suicidal ideation (Heffer & Willoughby, 2017). Table 4.1 gives a partial list of healthy coping skills that can be used to manage emotions and respond to conflict, grouped by their intended effects.

Table 4.1. Partial List of Coping Skills by Intended Effects

Self-Soothing Techniques that use the five senses to comfort yourself	Distraction Techniques that can help you take your mind off of your problems	Grounding and Mindfulness Techniques that help you focus on your present reality and get out of distressing thought patterns	Emotional Understanding Techniques to help yourself recognize and express your feelings
• Listening to music • Aromatherapy • Holding comforting objects • Massaging your hands or temples • Looking at pleasant images • Eating or drinking something tasty	• Reading a book • Watching TV or movies • Exercising • Spending time with friends • Cleaning or doing housework • Artwork and crafts	• Meditation • Breathing exercises • Yoga • Progressive muscle relaxation • Body scans	• Reviewing a chart of emotions • Journaling or writing • Drawing or painting • Dancing or movement • Speaking to someone • Asking yourself questions

Prior to reading the book, students can review this chart to familiarize themselves with examples of healthy coping. As an additional jigsaw activity, small groups of students can choose or be assigned a specific coping skill to research and present to the class. As students engage in their reading of the novel, they can draw upon their knowledge of these skills to help them identify whether the characters in the story are coping with the stressors they experience in healthy ways.

Expectations, Internal Conflict, and External Conflict

As teachers introduce the ideas of internal and external conflict, they can use a prompt focusing on what students may expect to find in the book: "Based on the title, *I Am Not Your Perfect Mexican Daughter*, what expectations or conflicts do you imagine that the protagonist, Julia, might face in the story?" As a class brainstorm, students can work to identify what the expectations of a "perfect" daughter might be, as well as identify indicators that a child might fall short of these expectations. As the group brainstorm takes place, teachers or students can document expectations onto post-it notes or index cards. The class can then sort the index cards based on whether the expectation in question

Table 4.2. Example Expectations Based on the Book Title

Based on the title I Am Not Your Perfect Mexican Daughter, what expectations do you imagine the protagonist, Julia, might face in the story?

Expectations of a "perfect" Mexican daughter	Obedient	Attends church
	Speaks Spanish	Gets good grades
	Keeps her room clean	Doesn't date
	Polite	Doesn't get in trouble
	Knows how to cook Mexican food	Doesn't use drugs or alcohol
	Helps with chores at home	Has polite friends

would indicate an internal conflict, external conflict, or combination of the two and support their hypothesis. Table 4.2 features examples of potential expectations reading.

As students continue reading the book, they can reflect on whether their expectations of conflict match or differ from what they read in the text. Journal entries or weekly writing exercises on this topic can help students explore character development and conflict related to characters' expectations and living realities. This activity can also connect to the "Reflecting on Mixed Identities" activity described later in this chapter to further explore how expectations and realities shift in different social contexts.

Preparing Students to Discuss Latinx Culture and Immigration

Julia is a Mexican American teenager with parents who immigrated to the United States illegally. They live in an area of Chicago that is heavily populated by other Mexican and Latinx people (a non-gendered alternative to "Latino" or "Latina"). Many of Julia's friends and classmates are Mexican American, and as such, the story draws upon Mexican and Latinx cultural norms. Readers will find that the book uses Spanish words and terms throughout, such as referring to Julia's parents as *Amá* and *Apá* instead of as *Mom* and *Dad*. Teachers should take preparatory steps such as having a Spanish-English dictionary or translation app available to help students identify and explore unfamiliar Spanish vocabulary.

It is impossible to discuss Mexican American culture without also discussing the role of immigration and the means by which Latinx people arrive in the United States. The immigrant experience is a key plot point in *I Am Not Your Perfect Mexican Daughter* as a major source of conflict and character development for Julia's mother and, by extension, for Julia and other members of the Reyes family. The book describes multiple betrayals by a "coyote," or smuggler, that involve rape, robbery, abandonment, and, in some cases, the death of immigrants attempting to cross the border (chapters 5, 22). These risks are common realities for immigrants attempting to cross into the United States. Undocumented immigrants are often negatively portrayed in news media and in politicized discussions, with a focus on the "illegal" nature of their arrival and representation as criminals attempting to subvert American economies and systems. These assertions, however, are untrue about the overwhelming majority of Mexican and Latinx immigrants, who often risk or experience serious trauma, harm, and financial hardship in their countries of origin, along their journeys, and after their arrival in the United States (Phipps & Degges-White, 2014).

Prior to reading the text, teachers can use additional media to familiarize students with various perspectives on the immigrant experience, and with contemporary portrayals of Mexican American culture, ensuring the inclusion of first-person perspectives. Doing so can help readers understand the cultural references throughout the book, increase empathy for the experience of the characters, and provide necessary context for the events that transpire in the novel. We offer a selection of potential resources in table 4.3, although there are certainly many other media sources available that explore the multifaceted Mexican American, Latinx, and immigrant experiences.

GUIDING STUDENTS THROUGH THE TEXT

Reflecting on Mixed Identities

Throughout the book, Julia finds that her sense of self is, at times, in conflict with her environment and with the expectations of others. Culturally, she finds herself split. Her Mexican-born family, her Mexican American friends, and the American school and city in which she lives all have different expectations of and priorities for her, and Julia struggles to find a singular, unified sense of herself. Drawing on the pre-reading activity that introduced internal and external conflict, students

Table 4.3. Resources for Contemporary Portrayals of Mexican American Culture

Resource	Summary
Name: *Ice El Hielo* Author: La Santa Cecilia (band) Format: music video (4 min., 29 sec.) Publication date: 2013	A music video for a Spanish-language song with lyrics and visual narratives sharing stories about the daily lives of undocumented Latinx immigrants, the constant fear they feel about the threat of being detained and deported by ICE, and the fractures caused to families by separation.
Name: *Mireya's Third Crossing* Author: Darcy Courteau Format: magazine article (*Atlantic*) Publication date: June 2019	Article detailing the real-life experience of a Mexican immigrant woman and her efforts to obtain permanent residency in the United States after living as an undocumented immigrant in Arkansas for more than 25 years. Describes the traumatic experiences she faces while crossing the border, her motives for coming to/staying in the United States, and the labor and financial burdens necessary to obtain a visa.
Name: *Gentefied* Author: Marvin Lemus and Linda Yvette Chávez (series creators) Format: television series (Netflix, approx. 30 min. episodes) Year: 2020	Television series following a Mexican American family living in the quickly gentrifying Boyle Heights neighborhood of Los Angeles. Addresses themes of Mexican/Latinx cultural identity, intergenerational cultural differences, the effects of gentrification on low-income and culturally marginalized neighborhoods, and the threat to Latinx people from law enforcement and ICE.
Name: *El Norte* Author: Gregory Nava (director) Format: film (2 hr., 21 min.) Year: 1983	Academy Award–winning Spanish-language film following two Guatemalan siblings who decide to leave their village after experiencing government-sanctioned violence and attempt the trek north to the United States. The film portrays the dangerous journey, including manipulation and violence by "coyotes," the motives for leaving one's home, and the discrepancy between the fantasy of the "American Dream" and the reality of life for undocumented immigrants.
Name: *La Frontera: El viaje con papá ~ My Journey with Papa* Authors: Deborah Mills and Alfredo Alva Format: picturebook Year: 2018	Illustrated bilingual (Spanish-English) children's picturebook following the journey of Alfredo and his father, who migrate from La Ceja in Guanajuato, Mexico, to the United States. The story includes a depiction of a "Coyote," who is named for the animal "known for its stealthy, wily ways," who helps them cross the border without documentation.

can use the following graphic organizer (see table 4.4), completed in full as an example, to define Julia's contextually dependent identities; recognize the impact of family, culture, and friends on her development; and consider how these differing identities contribute to Julia's internal and external conflicts.

Table 4.4. "Who Julia Is . . ." Sample Graphic Organizer for Julia's Various Identities

Who Julia is . . .	
To her family	Disrespectful and vulgar (chs. 1, 2, 13, 15, 23)
	Too "Americanized" (chs. 2, 3, 6, 13, 21–23)
	Ungrateful and spoiled (chs. 3, 5, 6, 9, 13)
	Untrustworthy (chs. 2, 7, 11, 14–16)
At school	A troublemaker (chs. 1, 3)
	A good writer with academic potential (chs. 3, 8, 14, 16, 28)
	Having a hard time and needs help/support (chs. 9, 10, 16, 18, 23)
	Can use her second-generation status as an academic advantage (ch. 14)
To her friends	Exaggerative (chs. 5, 10, 12, 25, 27)
	Sexually inexperienced (chs. 5, 10, 15)
	Thinks she's "better than everybody" and judgmental (chs. 9, 10, 12, 15)
	Considered pretty (chs. 10, 13, 15, 27)
To the world	Pitiable because of Olga's death (chs. 3, 7, 10, 14, 26)
	Delicate and sensitive (chs. 4, 7, 8, 17, 21)
	A snoop and a troublemaker (chs. 3, 4, 11, 12, 24–26)
	Too "brown" to be American and too American to fit in with her Mexican culture (chs. 1, 5, 14, 21, 25)
Really	Ambitious (chs. 1, 14, 15, 17, 19, 27)
(on the inside)	Unsure of how to express her feelings (chs. 1, 3, 11, 15–18, 22, 24, 27)
	Misses her sister and feels guilty about her death (chs. 1, 2, 13, 15, 17)
	Loves reading, art, eating, and writing (chs. 1, 2, 3, 5, 11, 14–16)
	Unhappy (chs. 11, 15, 16, 17, 22)
	Self-conscious about her body, cultural background, and poverty (chs. 2, 3, 5, 9, 13–15, 17, 19)

Debating Distance and Silence in the Context of Transgenerational Trauma

Silence and secrecy are pervasive themes that affect communication and cause conflict between many characters in the book: Olga's secrets lead to tension between Julia and her parents, Amá and Apá's secrecy about their experiences crossing the border create fears and strict rules for their daughters and lead both girls to keep secrets about their social activities and relationships. Moreover, Julia's difficulty communicating her feelings about Olga's death with others causes deep internal distress. In some of these cases, secrecy and silence benefit the secret-keeper and reduce external conflict, but they may also lead to increased external and internal conflict. Toward the end of the book in chapter 24, Julia confronts her sister's friend, Angie, about keeping Olga's pregnancy a secret even after Olga's death. Two perspectives become evident as

Angie says, "'Maybe you're too young to understand, Julia, but some-times people don't need the truth'" (p. 294), while Julia justifies her inquiry later by responding, "'I deserve to know. Because I, apparently, had no idea who Olga was. I guess none of us did.'" (p. 295).

A classroom debate centered on the question "Is it okay to keep secrets? If so, when and why?" will allow students to examine the risks and benefits of secrecy and silence, and identify how these tenden-cies exacerbate or reduce conflict—even within the context of shared trauma. Students will also consider how secrecy and openness affect how characters develop within the story. In "pro-" and "anti-"secrecy groups, students would first work to develop a thesis in response to this question, using the following sentence as a frame: "It is (not) okay to keep secrets because . . ." They would then work as groups to identify textual evidence using character statements or quotes from the book to support this thesis statement, and the teacher would facilitate a debate structured as follows:

1. Twenty minutes for debate preparation
2. Two minutes for affirmative ("yes") group's opening argument
3. Two minutes for negative ("no") group's opening argument
4. Two minutes for affirmative group to disagree
5. Two minutes for negative group to explain position
6. Ten-minute break for rebuttal and closing preparation
7. Two minutes for negative summary/rebuttal
8. Two minutes for affirmative summary/rebuttal

Students can link their debate considerations back to the "Who Julia is . . ." graphic organizer activity, referencing the ways in which Julia's identities are divided, depending on the cultural and social expectations she faces. It would also be worthwhile for students to consider secrecy and silence as specific responses to transgenerational trauma.

Exploring the Epitext: Author Q&A and Reading Group Guide

At the end of the novel, readers will find a Q&A with author Erika L. Sánchez, as well as a Reading Group Guide created by Maribel Castro.

The Reading Group Guide follows the chronology of the story, posing questions about specific scenes. These discussion questions address the many conflicting emotions and cultural/familial obligations facing Julia. Specifically, the thought-provoking questions invite readers to consider whether Julia's feelings, actions, and experiences are "right," "wrong," "reasonable," or "fair." Additionally, the Reading Group Guide walks readers through Julia's, and her family's, responses to pain, the secrets they keep from each other, and how it is (and is not) possible for them to fulfill their dreams in (or beyond) the United States. Teachers can use this epitext as an additional resource for centering discussions on character development and conflict.

Discussion Questions

Along with the epitext, teachers can use the following questions to address character development and the internal and external conflicts present in the story. These can be used to start individual writing prompts or guide small-group or class-wide discussions:

- What coping skills do Julia and other characters use in the story? How do these coping skills help or hurt the characters?
- What internal conflicts does Julia face, and what external conflicts does she face?
- How does the trauma of losing Olga directly affect Julia, Amá, and Apá? How does this trauma affect their relationships with each other and with other characters in the story?
- What conflicts (oppositional forces) do the characters, aside from Julia, face in the story? Have these characters experienced traumas that lead to conflict?
- How does Julia change from the beginning of the story, which opens with Olga's funeral, to the end, when she leaves Chicago for New York City to go to college?
- Why do characters like Lorena respond to Julia's unhappiness as they do? Are their responses to Julia justified (chapter 12)?
- How does Julia's experience of Mexican culture (including her experiences in the United States and in Mexico) influence her character development?

- Is Julia escaping from conflict by moving to New York City? If so, how? From what conflicts is Julia unable to escape?
- Is Julia done dealing with her and her family's traumas at the end of the book? What evidence supports your opinion?
- How do you imagine Julia's relationship with her parents will change in the future?

GUIDING STUDENTS OUT OF THE TEXT

A Call to Action

Throughout the book, Julia and other characters struggle with sharing the difficulties of their lives: depression and anxiety, trauma, abuse, relationships, and pregnancy, just to name a few. As students analyze the conflicts that arise within the book—many of which can be linked to transgenerational trauma and related behaviors, like keeping pain bottled up inside—teachers can help students consider, first, how secrecy and silence prolong and aggravate personal struggles and, second, how disclosure, even if painful, can lead to healing. The strategies that follow offer ways to help students break out of stigmatizing cultures of silence and make space to accept and support themselves and each other through moments of hardship.

Revising the Story

In chapter 12, Julia is hanging out with her best friend Lorena when she suddenly feels "sadness spreading inside" her and confides in her narration that she never knows "what to do when this happens" (p. 144). When Lorena asks her what's wrong, Julia confides that she hates her life and at times wishes she were dead. This moment, in retrospect, serves as a warning sign that Julia is having suicidal thoughts and is trying to seek support and validation from her friend. Yet Lorena responds angrily, slapping her on the arm and saying, "'Jesus, Julia. What the fuck? How can you say that?'" (p. 144). In pairs or small groups, students can practice empathy and imagine providing support to individuals who share that they are struggling by writing a script to revise this scene between Lorena and Julia. As guidance to writing, educators can pose questions such as the following:

1. How could Lorena have responded more supportively to Julia?
2. What action steps could Lorena and Julia take to make sure Julia receives help?
3. What resources or information might help Lorena and Julia address the situation more effectively?

Students may draw on their coping skill chart and the information they gathered during the trauma jigsaw pre-reading activity to inform their revisions. Role playing these revised scenes in class can also help students practice empathic responses to one another and learn varied supportive approaches by watching their peers in action. Since revising the scene calls for practicing both empathy and coping skills intended to provide support, it is recommended that this activity is done in collaboration with the school's mental health professional.

A Letter of Self-Acceptance

In the final chapters, Julia reflects on the various changes that have taken place in her life since Olga's death and since her own suicide attempt. She recognizes new coping skills she is using and acknowledges that sharing her thoughts and feelings with Dr. Cooke, Mr. Ingman, and her parents has been helpful in recovering from depression and in making her feel accepted for who she "really" is. At the very end of the book, Julia is on a plane, about to arrive in New York City and begin college all on her own, and in the final passage of the book, she shares, "These last two years I combed and delved through my sister's life to better understand her, which meant I learned how to find pieces of myself—both beautiful and ugly" (p. 340). Through the painful events and discoveries she has endured, Julia reaches a point of self-acceptance.

To reinforce student understanding of character development and recovery from trauma, they can engage in a letter-writing activity from the perspective of Julia writing to herself on the airplane, acknowledging her experiences of the past two years. The letter should state the events that Julia has endured and both name and validate the emotional reactions she had to them. The letter should also describe a minimum of three behavioral and emotional changes Julia has made from the start of the book to the end, remind Julia of healthy coping skills she can use as she begins college, and identify two hopes for herself as she enters this next phase of her life.

Closing the Book

Julia experiences various forms of primary and secondary trauma, and she has endured long periods of deep depression. While Julia struggles with trauma and depression related to familial death, her parents' trauma histories, bicultural pressures, and more throughout the book, at a critical point she receives care and support and begins to heal from her experiences. As students finish their work with this text, they should be able to identify the damaging effects of secrecy on Julia and other characters, identify the benefits of receiving support, and name healthy coping skills to manage distress.

To demonstrate understanding of trauma and its effects, students can engage in a public awareness campaign and spread the knowledge they have gained. Classes can revisit previously established community partnerships with public health officials, university or college professors, or local mental health providers to host an event for the school or in the local community. Returning to the original jigsaw groups, students can create pamphlets or posters that can be shared to provide education and resources on trauma to members of the community outside of the classroom. These visual aids could be shared in school hallways, or at a table in a school fair where mental health professionals from the school or community are available to provide additional information or support if needed.

As an in-class activity that connects the mental health knowledge back to the book, the jigsaw groups' posters could be displayed around the classroom for a Gallery Walk, through which students would read and respond to each other's work (with sticky notes, if desired), linking to moments in the text where this specific trauma concept is found. Students can also write positive messages in chalk around their school and/or neighborhood, using words and phrases to encourage others to accept growth, like Julia, and recognize that hardship is common but is something we can all learn to cope with.

CONCLUSION

Most characters in *I Am Not Your Perfect Mexican Daughter* have faced hardship, trauma, or loss. Many people in the world have similar experiences, but discussing these issues is not often the norm. Throughout her book, Sánchez shows readers how common secrecy and silence occur in response to trauma, and how serious the consequences of silence can be. In exploring Julia's experience as a teenage girl struggling with grief, while being pulled between the cultural expectations of her family, her friends, and society, readers can see how trauma and silence leave Julia struggling without access to support and resources. In her Q&A at the end of the book, Sánchez shares that she wants her readers to know that "teens often struggle with mental illness and need help: therapy, medication, etc. I want young readers to know that they're not alone and that life can get better" (p. 347). As readers explore the character development of Julia and those surrounding her in *I Am Not Your Perfect Mexican Daughter*, as well as the internal and external conflicts present in the story, they are encouraged to recognize that trauma and hardship are normal human experiences, and that help and support are available. By opening ourselves to self-acceptance as Julia does, which sometimes requires revealing secrets buried within, one is able to begin the journey toward healing.

REFERENCES

American Psychiatric Association. (2013). *Diagnostic and statistical manual of mental disorders* (5th ed.). Washington, DC: American Psychiatric Publishing. https://doi.org/10.1176/appi.books.9780890425596

Centers for Disease Control. (2020, December 2). *Anxiety and depression in children: Get the facts.* https://www.cdc.gov/childrensmentalhealth/features/anxiety-depression-children.html

Corless, I. B., Limbo, R., Bousso, R. S., Wrenn, R. L., Head, D., Lickiss, N., & Wass, H. (2014). Languages of grief: A model for understanding the expressions of the bereaved. *Health Psychology and Behavioral Medicine, 2*(1), 132–43. https://doi.org/10.1080/21642850.2013.879041

Dutro, E. (2019). *The vulnerable heart of literacy: Centering trauma as powerful pedagogy.* New York: Teachers College Press.

Heffer, T,. & Willoughby, T. (2017). A count of coping strategies: A longitudinal study investigating an alternative method to understanding coping and adjustment. *PLoS One, 12*(10), e0186057. https://doi.org/10.1371/journal.pone.0186057

Peña, J. B., Wyman, P. A., Brown, C. H., Matthieu, M. M., Olivares, T. E., Hartel, D., & Zayas, L. H. (2008). Immigration generation status and its association with suicide attempts, substance use, and depressive symptoms among Latino adolescents in the USA. *Prevention Science, 9*(4), 299–310. https://doi.org/10.1007%2Fs11121-008-0105-x

Phipps, R. M., & Degges-White, S. (2014). A new look at transgenerational trauma transmission: Second-generation Latino immigrant youth. *Journal of Multicultural Counseling and Development, 42*(3), 174–87. https://doi.org/10.1002/j.2161-1912.2014.00053.x

Sánchez, E. L. (2017). *I am not your perfect Mexican daughter.* New York: Knopf.

Stone, D. M., Holland, K. M., Bartholow, B., Crosby, A. E., Davis, S., & Wilkins, N. (2017). *Preventing suicide: A technical package of policies, programs, and practices.* Atlanta, GA: National Center for Injury Prevention and Control, Centers for Disease Control and Prevention.

Telzer, E. H., van Hoorn, J., Rogers, C. R., & Do, K. T. (2018). Chapter seven: Social influence on positive youth development: A developmental neuroscience perspective. *Advances in Child Development and Behavior, 54,* 215–58. https://doi.org/10.1016/bs.acdb.2017.10.003

Trauma and Learning Policy Initiative. (2013). *Helping traumatized children learn 2: Creating and advocating for trauma-sensitive schools.* Boston and Cambridge: Massachusetts Advocates for Children and Harvard Law School.

5

EXPLORING GRAPHIC MEMOIR TRAJECTORIES

Processing the Effects of Substance Use Disorder and Healing through Art in *Hey, Kiddo*

Grace Enriquez and Michelle Pate

Every family looks different, and every family has its own strengths and challenges. While some children live with a mother and father or maybe two mothers or fathers, or just one parent, others might be adopted. Still others may live with grandparents, aunts, or uncles, or in a foster home. Regardless of what one's family looks like, substance use disorder (SUD) can affect anyone and anywhere. *Hey, Kiddo,* the National Book Award finalist graphic memoir by Jarrett Krosoczka (2018) chronicles the impact of addiction on a family.

Substance use disorder is defined as "recurrent use of alcohol or other drugs (or both)" that results in significant impairment in several areas, including employment, relationships, and finances (Lipari & Van Horn, 2017, p. 1). Based upon survey data collected through the National Surveys on Drug Use and Health (Lipari & Van Horn, 2017), as many as "1 in 8 children (8.7 million) aged 17 or younger lived in households with at least one parent who had a past year substance use disorder" (p. 1). Research has shown that children of parents with SUD were often found to be of lower socioeconomic status and had more difficulties in academic, social, and family functioning when compared with children of parents who do not have substance use disorder (Peleg-Oren & Teichman, 2006). These children are also more likely to have higher rates of mental and behavioral disorders (Peleg-Oren & Teichman, 2006). Additionally, children who are exposed to a parent with SUD are more likely to develop SUD symptoms themselves (Lipari & Van Horn, 2017).

This chapter will guide teachers and students through Krosoczka's graphic memoir as he uses art to heal and process his mother's struggles with substance use disorder. Specifically, this chapter highlights the unique qualities of plot in memoir and visual storytelling in graphic format. With this lens, students can explore how the trajectories of plot and graphic storytelling provide an honest depiction of the complexities of a family impacted by substance use disorder.

UNDERSTANDING SUD IN THE CONTEXT OF ADDICTION

Addiction, also known as dependence, is an umbrella term that describes the behavior that is associated with disorders such as SUD, gambling, and alcoholism and is characterized as a mental health disorder that can affect thinking, behavior, and mood (Substance Abuse and Mental Health Services Administration [SAMHSA], 2019). Addiction is not something that an individual chooses; rather, it comprises a complex mixture of genetic and environmental factors such as brain chemistry, inherited traits, and environmental exposure (Doweiko, 2009). Addiction can affect anyone regardless of socioeconomic status, education, race, gender, or other demographics. But many of these characteristics can increase the severity of addiction to alcohol, non-prescribed pharmaceuticals, and illicit drugs.

Although Krosoczka describes several types of addiction in his memoir, including alcohol and tobacco, this chapter focuses on his mother's addiction to illicit drugs, more specifically heroin, indicating a substance use disorder. Addiction is complex; therefore, the effects can be long lasting and impactful not only for people diagnosed with SUD but also for their families. Long-term health effects of SUD can include heart, kidney, and liver damage, while long-term cognitive effects can include memory loss, impaired decision making and processing, and loss of brain cells over time (Doweiko, 2009). Children who remain in the care of someone with a SUD can be at higher risk for neglect and abuse, instances of depression and anxiety, and developing SUD symptoms (SAMHSA, 2019).

HEY, KIDDO BY JARRETT KROSOCZKA

As a young child, Jarrett moves in with his maternal grandparents, unsure of where his mother is going, why his grandparents are adopting him, or the identity of his father. As Jarrett grows up, his mother Leslie periodically reappears in his life through letters and the occasional surprise visit. Just as soon as they reconnect, she disappears again. Ultimately, Jarrett's adolescence and life trajectory are shaped by his grandparents, whose loud presence and immense love provide the strength he needs to realize and come to terms with Leslie's addiction to heroin. It is through their support that Jarrett takes his first drawing class and launches himself on a profound personal and professional journey toward acceptance and healing.

GUIDING STUDENTS INTO THE TEXT

Mental Health Literacy

Addiction often remains hidden in the shadows and may be kept as a family secret. This is the case in *Hey, Kiddo* as Jarrett's family attempts to shield him from his mother's SUD and other addictive behaviors. This is also prevalent in his writing as often the diagnosis or acknowledgment of a SUD is frequently characterized by behaviors that result from Leslie's drug use such as stealing, arrests, and overdosing. Although this chapter focuses on addressing Jarrett's mother's substance abuse, other themes may arise for students when reading this memoir, such as living with a single parent, teen pregnancy, teen alcohol use, and loss. The theme of loss is woven throughout *Hey, Kiddo*, as Jarrett repeatedly experiences the loss of his mother as she transitions in and out of his life and ultimately dies as a consequence of her substance use disorder.

Outlined here are common terms referenced in the book that can help students discuss and understand substance use disorder. In understanding these terms, students can articulate the known mental health concepts and associated factors prevalent throughout the novel.

- *Drug addict:* A drug addict is a person addicted to using illegal drugs (SAMHSA, 2019). Although the term *drug addict* is only used in chapter 4, the defining behaviors are present throughout the book.

  - It is important to note that the term *drug addict* labels individuals by their actions; in the mental health field using the phrase "person who is addicted to drugs" is preferred as this identifies the person first instead of their actions or diagnosis (Atayde et al., 2021).

- *Alcohol use disorder (AUD):* Alcohol use disorder, or alcoholism, is a pattern of alcohol use that impacts several areas of an individual's life negatively, for example, health, social relationships, employment (SAMHSA, 2019), (chapters 3 and 4). AUD is considered a medical condition and can be categorized as mild, moderate, or severe.
- *Substance use disorder (SUD):* Substance use disorder is a pattern of continued use despite negative consequences of drugs, alcohol, or a combination that results in significant impairment in several areas, including employment, relationships, and finances (Lipari & Van Horn, 2017), (chapters 4 and 5).

  - Substance use disorder and the negative consequences can be read throughout the memoir. Some instances of these negative consequences are when Leslie steals a scarf from the mall and is then arrested (chapter 2) or how Leslie's relationship with her family—and, most important, her son Jarrett—is jeopardized by her SUD.

- *Relapse program:* A relapse program is often referred to as "rehab." These programs are intensive inpatient treatment facilities that often address the medical, physical, and emotional aspects of substance use disorder. They are addressed through doctor and nursing services; individual, group, and family therapy sessions; and relapse prevention plans (chapter 7).

- *Halfway home:* After completing a relapse program, participants may attend a halfway home, which is a less restrictive environment that allows individuals to build everyday living skills in a sober environment (chapter 5).
- *Ward of the state:* A child becomes a ward of the state when that child's parent/caregiver is no longer fit to parent the child and there are no other relatives who are fit and willing to care for the child. At that time, the child goes into the care of the state. This means that the parent/caregiver's rights can be taken away and the child will go to live in a foster home until the parent/caregiver is able to be deemed fit to care for the child or the child is adopted (chapter 1).
- *OD'ing:* "Overdosing," or "OD'ing," is when someone takes a toxic amount of one substance or a toxic amount of several substances at once. This often results in unconsciousness, slowed heart rate, labored breathing, and possibly death (chapter 6).
- *Art as therapy:* Often art can be used as a way to process difficult emotions and help relieve stress and anxiety (Edith & Gerity, 2000). This concept is prevalent throughout the memoir.

Principles of Graphic Novel/Memoir Illustration

In today's world, students are surrounded by texts that present information through various media and modalities. The ability to read illustrations is key to making sense of that information, as many of the texts that society consumes today are oriented or supported through images. Visual literacy is also a crucial skill needed to read graphic novels and memoir. As such, before reading *Hey, Kiddo*, teachers could first introduce students to principles of illustration (Bang, 2016), which explains how artists manipulate various elements of pictures to produce emotional responses in readers. Such elements include shape, space, line, color, light, size, and contrast. For example, a large shape in bold color placed in the center of the page conveys its importance, and a character drawn with rounded shapes and curves is more comforting than one drawn with sharp angles. How an illustrator uses and adjusts each of these elements can influence the reader's response and interpretation of the image.

Graphic storytellers apply these illustrative principles in a variety of ways through the specific text structure of a graphic novel or memoir. Teachers may want to introduce students to some additional terms and design elements important in graphic texts, such as panel (an individual segment of illustration and text), frame (the border of a segment), gutter (the space between frames and pages), bleed (an image that extends beyond a frame or page), caption (written text that provides narration or description), and speech/thought balloon (the enclosed words spoken or thought by a character) (ReadWriteThink, 2008).

Once students gain an understanding of these visual elements, teachers can direct them to examine the front cover and draw their attention to the colors: What do they notice about the kinds of blue that Krosoczka used? What message might he be sending through this visual? Next, teachers can ask students to take a look at the posture (shape) Krosoczka used to draw his younger self: What might it convey about his character? From there, teachers can ask students to examine other elements, especially the use of light and dark, to elicit more predictions about the memoir. Students can contrast the front cover illustration with the illustration on the very first page of the book, in which Jarrett illustrates himself as a young child. They can then do the same with the next page of the book, the illustrated title page, the copyright, and dedication pages, using the illustration principles to elicit and deepen their predictions about the story.

Using these illustration principles, teachers can guide students through the rest of the memoir as they preview the pages, or do a "picture walk," to gather a sense of the rest of the illustrations. Students can take note of what they notice about Krosoczka's illustration style and how it supports their predictions. Specifically, students can focus on the pages where Krosoczka changes the medium and style, such as the chapter dividers. Why might he have incorporated such changes? How do the visual images support any prediction students might have about what will happen next in the story, or enhance their understanding of the chapters they have already read? Additionally, teachers might want students to consider the full-page wedding dance (p. 23), the various nightmare scenes (pp. 48–49, 78–79, 124), the disclosure of Leslie's addiction (pp. 134–35), and the full-page wordless scene in which Jarrett draws a self-portrait (p. 233).

Contemplating the Peritext

Krosoczka bookends the story he wants to tell with additional text and images before and after the main narrative. This peritextual material supplements the central text. Students may be familiar with the ways a prologue, epilogue, author's/illustrator's note, and other front and back matter in a book can extend their understanding of the main text; however, graphic texts are increasingly making use of the book cover, endpapers, dedication page, copyright page, title page, and other such peritexts to support the central text (Sipe, 2011).

Teachers can ask students to consider the peritext of *Hey, Kiddo* by closely examining the words and images included. Specifically, teachers can point out the full-page illustrations placed before the title page and the double-page spreads that encompass the title page, dedication page, and each chapter break. Students can examine the words and images on those pages to predict what will happen in the main narrative. They can also study the photographs of notes from Jarrett's grandparents and mother that appear at the end of the book, as well as the photograph of the book in manuscript form. Teachers also might want to point out the recurring pineapple print in the background of these pages to draw students' attention to how motifs might be threaded throughout graphic novels and memoir plots to signify a certain theme.

Three-Way Dialogue Journals

Given the complex and personal nature of SUD, students may have questions and reflections they are not comfortable sharing in front of the class. Teachers can partner with the school's and/or district's student support team (school psychologist, guidance counselor, social worker, etc.) to provide a confidential, knowledgeable sounding board for students. Students can maintain dialogue journals with the teacher and one support team staff member, where they write their questions and reflections to share in a one-to-one written conversation. While it may be helpful on occasion to offer prompts to motivate student writing, the chief purpose of this activity is to encourage students to use writing as a way to engage in meaningful contemplation and inquiry about SUD or the plot and character development in the memoir. Teachers should keep in mind that this activity is not intended to position the teacher as a counselor or therapist; rather, dialogue journals are a space to gather information about students' prior knowledge and questions, as well as to promote further research and understanding about the information they may have acquired elsewhere. Since this is a three-way dialogue journal, the school's support team colleague should be the one to address any questions that fall outside of the teacher's expertise and qualifications as a classroom teacher. Some prompts the teacher might offer when a student seems reluctant to write could include the following:

- What prior knowledge do you have about substance use disorder? What books, movies, or other sources have contributed to your knowledge about substance use disorder?
- Why might the causes and effects of SUD reach beyond an individual person?
- What resources does your school or local community provide to learn about and deal with substance use disorder?

Students should be encouraged, rather than assigned, to answer such questions, and they should do so only if they feel comfortable. Students can also be encouraged to ask any question and write their honest thoughts about SUD, without fear of being judged or the pressure of being assessed on their writing skills. These journals are not meant to assess students' reading comprehension; rather, their purpose is to promote dialogue about SUD and the way it is portrayed in this graphic memoir.

GUIDING STUDENTS THROUGH THE TEXT

Making Sense of Complex Plot Structures

In the English language arts class, students learn that narrative plots follow an arc or mountain structure. Real life, however, doesn't always comply with a progressive arc of events. The plot of *Hey, Kiddo* follows more of a mountain range rather than a single mountain, with several series of events that gain momentum toward a narrative climax and resolution before moving on to the next. To help readers make sense of this

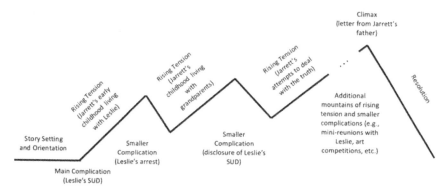

Figure 5.1. Mountain Range Plot Structure of *Hey, Kiddo*

plot structure, teachers can support the mountain range analogy with a graphic organizer similar to figure 5.1.

Another analogy that can help students grasp the concept of multiple subplots within a single overall narrative is that of ocean waves moving toward the shore. Rather than putting all its energy into creating a single wave, the momentum of the plot rises and falls as a series of connected crests and troughs that eventually crest and break. Just as waves become taller as they approach the shore, the action swells and drops in smaller sizes at first and then builds toward a more substantial narrative climax. The breaking waves analogy can be supported with a graphic organizer similar to the one in figure 5.2 and adapted to accommodate as many wave crests and troughs as needed. While the exact number of crests and troughs can make for an engaging debate among students through a close reading of the plot, teachers can anticipate at least eight sets of crests and troughs.

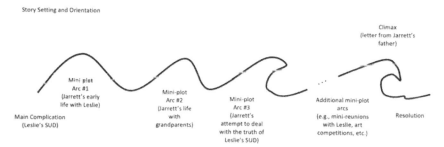

Figure 5.2. Breaking Waves Plot Structure of *Hey, Kiddo*

Approaching the plot of *Hey, Kiddo* as a mountain range or breaking waves can help students highlight Jarrett's character development. After initially framing the novel as a flashback in the prologue, chapter 1 begins tracing his family's story beginning with his grandparents' courtship and struggles to secure a financial footing for their growing family and ending with Jarrett's birth. Chapter 2 describes what Jarrett remembers about his early years living with Leslie, and chapter 3 details life with his grandparents after they assume guardianship. Here, readers can see the plot rising and falling in small increments. Brief moments, such as Jarrett's first reunion with his mother at the halfway house, form the early, smaller mountains or waves as the excitement builds and then subsides. When Jarrett's grandparents reveal the truth about his mother's SUD, chapter 4 provides another small climax that propels the overall narrative arc forward. In chapter 5, the focus shifts a bit to Jarrett's burgeoning talent as an artist, culminating in his first published work: the cover of his eighth-grade yearbook. The plot continues in this manner through the remaining chapters, with his mother's visits remaining unpredictable and his artistic development growing, leading to an unexpected reunion with his father.

As students track the plot trajectory using a graphic organizer (see table 5.1 as an example), they can come to see how each mini-arc, mountain, or wave corresponds with Jarrett's development. Each reunion with his mother brings about another round of expectation, excitement, and adjustment to the reality that Jarrett must learn to navigate. Each event in his grandparents' home or with his peers helps explain how and why Jarrett gravitated toward art and eventually pursued it as a career. Each encounter in his art classes impacts his ability to establish something stable and rewarding in his daily life. Using a graphic organizer in this way not only can help students make sense of a complex plot but also helps them make sense of the character's progression in his thoughts, feelings, and worldview from childhood to adolescence and ultimately to adulthood.

Exploring the Complex Causes of SUD

The root causes of SUD stem from a combination of genetic and environmental factors. Krosoczka portrays this combination throughout

Table 5.1. Cheat Sheet of Key Plot Points in *Hey, Kiddo*

Chapter	Key Plot Points
Prologue	Jarrett practices driving with Joe in a cemetery. They discuss where the Krosoczka family is and will be buried one day.
1: Family History	Jarrett narrates the story of his grandparents' courtship, early days of marriage, and the growth of their family. He then tells the story of how his parents met, how his father abandoned his pregnant mother (Leslie), and how he was born.
2: Life with Leslie	Jarrett shares some memories of his early childhood years living with Leslie, both the good and the bad. His nightmares begin. Leslie is arrested, and Joe and Shirley (his grandparents) become Jarrett's legal guardians.
3: Skipping a Generation	Jarrett describes life with his grandparents and the occasional visits with and letters from Leslie. He meets a new friend, Pat, and continues having nightmares.
4: Disclosure	Jarrett's grandparents reveal the truth about Leslie's substance use disorder.
5: Pen to Paper	Joe enrolls Jarrett, now in middle school, in art classes. Jarrett continues seeing Leslie occasionally. He graduates from middle school and has his artwork published on the cover of his school's yearbook.
6: Hard Work	Jarrett is bullied in high school but finds solace in art class. His drawings catch his teachers' attention for better or worse, and he wins a citywide newspaper editorial cartoon contest. Jarrett begins working in Joe's factory but is encouraged by his aunt to become an artist instead.
7: Ghosts	Jarrett uses art to deal with everyday events in high school and at home. Leslie returns home for Christmas with a new boyfriend. Jarrett gets a letter from his father.
8: Lost and Found	Jarrett applies to art school. He has his first honest conversation with Leslie, and he meets his father and stepsiblings. Jarrett graduates from high school and reflects on his family.

the book, showing both the evidence of SUD in his grandparents, the family, and social scenes that possibly contributed to his mother's addiction. Readers see examples of the "strangers coming in and out of the house" (pp. 47–50) and the "terrible decisions" Leslie made, such as shoplifting and abetting violent behavior that "would forever alter our relationship as mother and son" (pp. 60–61). Readers see Jarrett's grandparents furiously arguing because some nights his grandfather "wouldn't come home at the end of the day. . . . Then the front door would open and the smell of alcohol would fill the house" (pp. 76–77). Both grandparents are also depicted throughout the book with a cigarette in hand or mouth.

Table 5.2. T-Chart Listing Genetic and Environmental Influences

Genetic Factors	Environmental Influences
Genetic influence	Parental substance abuse
Heredity	Lack of stability early in life
	Peer pressure
	Normalization of substance use

Before starting the activity, teachers can engage readers in examination of "genetic factors" and common "environmental influences" that can potentially lead to substance use disorder. Teachers can work alongside the school's mental health professional to facilitate the conversation and guide students through a discussion of nature versus nurture and how that speaks to their reading of the graphic memoir.

As teachers begin an examination of these factors within the text, they can use these examples as launching points for whole-class and small-group discussions about the complexities and causes of substance use disorder. Teachers can begin by having students create a table or T-chart listing genetic factors on one side and the environmental influences on the other as they relate to the protagonist within the memoir (see table 5.2).

As students move through the text, teachers can encourage them to consider how the influences shape each character's journey and impact plot development.

Genre Exploration: Memoir

As previously mentioned, *Hey, Kiddo* is a graphic memoir of Krosoczka's childhood and adolescence. Rather than catalog what happened from birth to present in an author's life, a memoir focuses on a certain memory or set of related memories that may consist of several events that occurred throughout a longer time span.

As students near the conclusion of their reading, they can take time to examine why *Hey, Kiddo* can be considered a memoir. To determine a focus of the main text, teachers might have students flip through the book, noting the chapter titles and reflecting upon their newfound understanding of the plot and characters' development from the illustrations and snippets of text. Teachers can then ask students to use that information to identify what parameters Krosoczka set for the part of his life story that he wanted to share. Students can use their responses to frame their reading of the memoir and build an initial understanding of the plot's progression.

To extend their understanding of this kind of plot structure, teachers might have students construct a list of related memories and events that they feel have defined their sense of self and understanding of the world thus far. Students can use this list to compose their own mini-memoirs, consisting of perhaps three or four of those memories and events, and applying what they have been learning about how such memories and events can be connected into a story of their lives. Finally, teachers might allow students to compose their mini-memoirs in the graphic format if that modality showcases their strengths as storytellers more than using only written text.

Discussion Questions

Reading *Hey, Kiddo* provides many opportunities for students to pause, dig deeper, and consider what the text reflects about the complexities of substance use disorder. The following are some questions to encourage further inquiry, close reading, and critical thinking about the book:

- Although the memoir revolves around Jarrett's abandonment by his mother, Jarrett begins retelling his family's history with his grandparents starting their life together as a family (pp. 14–41). Why might he have chosen that as a starting point? After reading the novel, consider the following question: How do Jarrett's grandparents contribute to the events that occur throughout the book and his childhood, for better or worse?
- Dreams can often be symbolic of our real-life thoughts, feelings, and concerns. What might Jarrett's nightmares symbolize? Who or what might the monsters represent? Why might Jarrett be unable to stop them in his dream? Consider the events Jarrett narrates before and after mentioning the nightmares. Refer to pp. 48–49, pp. 76–79.
- At different points after Jarrett moves in with his grandparents, Leslie reappears in his life for brief moments. How does Leslie's

SUD impact what they do and where they are during those re-
unions? What emotions do Jarrett, Leslie, and his grandparents
experience? What emotions do they express? Refer to pp. 82–84,
94–95, 156–59, 168–71.

- When Leslie gives Jarrett the stuffed bear, he reflects, "When you
  don't see your mom much, you treasure anything that she gives
  you" (p. 84). There are many examples of gift giving throughout
  Hey, Kiddo, such as when Jarrett's grandparents get him a hamster
  (pp. 110–11), when they surprise him with a trip to Disney World
  (pp. 128–29), when Leslie gives him a crystal (p. 159), and when
  Jarrett gives his grandparents a portrait he painted of them (pp.
  247–48). How might each gift say something about Jarrett's relationship with the gift giver or receiver?

- The dynamics in Jarrett's family are complicated. When Holly
  moves out, what do you think each family member is feeling? How
  does your knowledge of each character support your initial infer-
  ence? Refer to pp. 90–95.

- When Pat moves into the house next door, he and Jarrett become
  close friends. What characteristics and qualities does Pat have that
  seem helpful and supportive to Jarrett? How does their friendship
  provide support to Jarrett in a way that's different from the support
  of his family? What characteristics and qualities do you value in a
  friendship? Refer to pp. 102–16.

- When Jarett's grandparents finally reveal the truth of his mother's
  SUD and whereabouts, Jarrett states, "I knew in that moment,
  when my grandfather told me the plain truth, that life wouldn't be
  the same for me. It didn't change the circumstances, but it shifted
  my perspective" (p. 138). How so? What did Jarrett think and do
  differently when he talked about or interacted with his mother
  from that moment on? Refer to pp. 132–39.

- The high school art teacher, Mr. Shilale, tells students, "There is no
  such thing as a mistake, only a correction" (p. 197). How does this
  advice apply not just to Jarrett's art but also his approach to life?

- When he is a senior in high school, Jarrett finally expresses anger toward Leslie, declaring that Shirley is his mother. He also
  finally gets the opportunity to meet his biological father and his
  half-siblings. What do those interactions reveal about the growth

or development of each character—Jarrett, Leslie, and Richard—throughout the years? Refer to pp. 274–93.

GUIDING STUDENTS OUT OF THE TEXT

A Call to Action

Bringing Community Awareness

Now that students have learned about SUD and mental health, they can take action to educate others. One way teachers can accomplish this is to have students create posters or flyers that educate the community on SUD and mental health. This would be a great opportunity to pair with the school's art teacher, guidance counselor, and local law enforcement to discuss how information about SUD and mental health can be brought out into the public and reduce the stigma that is attached to both. These posters/flyers can serve as educational tools in schools and communities. Suggested materials to have available for students include thick cardstock paper (various colors and sizes), markers, crayons, colored pencils, paint, glue, and magazines. As students craft their posters, they should consider that SUD is not a choice, but a mental health diagnosis, and that SUD can happen to anyone despite race, ethnicity, socioeconomic status, or level of education. Most important, students should incorporate information concerning community organizations and resources that can support those in need. Finally, as students determine the visual representations they want to incorporate into their poster, they should be mindful of graphic images depicting drugs or drug use, as this may be triggering for anyone viewing the poster.

Front and Back Matter

After reading the memoir, teachers can have students revisit the prologue, author's note, and notes on the art. What kind of information does each provide? How does it supplement the main narrative? How did their reading of the text compare to their initial predictions and picture walk?

In a narrative story structure, a prologue can take many forms and serve different purposes. One purpose is to provide background information about events leading up to the main story line; in other words, it provides a setup for the story. Another purpose is to entice the reader with a clue or statement that will only make sense if one reads the main narrative. Sometimes prologues provide an alternative perspective, addressing the main events of the story to come from another point of view. Teachers can ask students to consider the following questions: What do you identify to be the purpose of Krosoczka's prologue? Why do you think he begins his memoir with a prologue, rather than start with the main story line? How does this approach enhance the themes and purpose of that main story line?

Likewise, the format and purpose of an author's note can differ. Sometimes, an author provides additional information about the places and people in the story, perhaps telling what happened after the events of the main narrative come to a resolution. Other times, an author will discuss the process of writing. Teachers can ask students to consider the following: What information does the author provide, and why might he include this information for the reader? How does his author's note support, challenge, or complicate your understanding of the main narrative and Jarrett's relationship with his family?

Authors may also include the additional back matter in a book, such as a glossary, time line, acknowledgments, and resources for further reading and learning related to the main narrative. As teachers bring the discussion of the plot to a close, they can have students consider these questions: What back matter material is included in *Hey, Kiddo*? How does that material further enhance your understanding of Jarrett's memoir?

Graphic Novel Practice

Now that students have explored the front and back matter of the memoir, teachers could address the art that was created to tell Jarrett's story. After writing this graphic memoir, Jarrett noted in "A Note on the Art" section, "Creating the art for this book has been the most profound artistic endeavor I have yet to undertake" (para. 6). This quote provides a great framework to have students demonstrate their understanding of the graphic novel structure. Using a graphic novel template, students could be given time, space, and materials to create a graphic novel about one of the supporting characters in the memoir. It might be best to engage the school's art teacher to assist students in their illustrations and use of lesser-known materials.

Closing the Book

Art as a Processing Tool

There are many benefits to creating art whether consciously or unconsciously. Drake et al. (2016) identify that art has the "power to improve mood" and "reduc[e] trauma-related symptoms" (p. 325), while Van Lith (2015) suggests that art can help relieve tension and unresolved feelings that can impact an individual on many levels. Jarrett uses art throughout his life as a way to process his past and escape the realities of being a child of a mother addicted to illicit drugs. In chapter 5, Krosoczka writes that when he creates comics he escapes into something he created because in the real world he doesn't have control of anything. Later in chapter 7, he identifies the additional ways in which he has used art throughout his life: to get attention, to impress people, and finally just to survive the ghosts of his past, which art has allowed him to face.

To conclude students' study of the text, teachers might ask if they have ever doodled when stressed or listened to music to ease some heavy feelings. After discussing how art can be of therapeutic value, teachers can encourage students to write or discuss in small groups how Jarrett uses art throughout the memoir, and how his art further develops his characters' identities. Although this memoir can potentially stir up mixed emotions for students, it is important for teachers to provide students with closure and allow them to process the text. One thing that lends itself to processing is art. Allowing students the time and space to create art can be an important outlet for mental health.

CONCLUSION

In his author's note, Krosoczka wrote, "It is said that books save lives, but I also say that empty sketchbooks save lives, too" (p. 305) *Hey, Kiddo* exemplifies how any form of art—from storytelling to illustration—can help address the challenges associated with substance use disorder. Krosoczka supports readers who are new to the topic by providing a multilayered representation of the daily experiences of a family impacted by substance use disorder. Perhaps, more important, he provides readers who are all too familiar with SUD a means to see the hopes and healing possibilities of art and illustration in their lives.

REFERENCES

Atayde, A., Hauc, S., Bessette, L., Danckers, H., & Saitz, R. (2021). Changing the narrative: A call to end stigmatizing terminology related to substance use disorders. *Addiction Research & Theory*, 1–4. https://doi.org/10.1080/16066 359.2021.1875215

Bang, M. (2016). *Picture this: How pictures work*. San Francisco, CA: Chronicle Books.

Doweiko, H. (2009). *Concepts of chemical dependency*. Boston, MA: Brooks/ Cole, Cengage Learning.

Drake, J., Hastedt, I., & James, C. (2016). Drawing to distract: Examining the psychological benefits of drawing over time. *Psychology of Aesthetics, Creativity, and the Arts*, 10(3), 325–31. https://doi.org/10.1037/aca0000064

Edith, K., & Gerity, L. (2000). *Art as therapy: Collected papers*. Jessica Kingsley.

Krosoczka, J. (2018). *Hey, kiddo*. New York: Graphix.

Lipari, R. N., & Van Horn, S. L. (2017). Children living with parents who have a substance use disorder. In *The CBHSQ Report* (pp. 1–7). Rockville, MD: Substance Abuse and Mental Health Services Administration.

Peleg-Oren, N., & Teichman, M. (2006). Young children of parents with substance use disorder (SUD): A review of literature and implications for social work practice. *Journal of Social Work Practice in the Addictions*, 6(1–2), 49–61. https://doi.org/10.1300/J160v06n01_03

ReadWriteThink. (2008). *Graphic novel/comics terms and concepts*. www.read writethink.org/files/resources/lesson_images/lesson1102/terms.pdf

Sipe, L. R. (2011). The art of the picturebook. In S. A. Wolf, K. Coats, P. Enciso, & C. A. Jenkins (Eds.), *Handbook of research on children's and young adult literature* (pp. 238–52). New York: Routledge.

Substance Abuse and Mental Health Services Administration. (2019). Center for behavioral health statistics and quality. National survey on drug use and health. Table 5.4B—Alcohol use disorder in past year among persons aged 12 or older, by age group and demographic characteristics: Percentages, 2018 and 2019. https://www.samhsa.gov/data/sites/default/files/re ports/rpt29394/NSDUHDetailedTabs2019/NSDUHDetTabsSect5pe2019 .htm?s=5.4&#tab5-4b

Van Lith, T. (2015). Art making as a mental health recovery tool for change and coping. *Art Therapy*, 32(1), 5–12. https://doi.org/10.1080/07421656 .2015.992826

6

TEACHING *WHEN REASON BREAKS*

Understanding Depression and Interrogating Bias through Character Analysis

Elsie Lindy Olan, Kia Jane Richmond, and Mary Mae Kelly

Reading books about young adults who exhibit symptoms of depression can be a gateway for teens (and adults) to develop a better understanding of—and empathy for—people potentially living with mental illness. Being sad as a teenager is part of the developmental process: we lose friends; we don't make the team; the person we are interested in doesn't like us back; we get grounded for making bad decisions; our parents fight or get divorced. There is a difference, however, between sadness, an emotional response to a troubling event or experience, and a clinical diagnosis of major depression with a risk of suicidal behavior. According to the *Diagnostic and Statistical Manual of Mental Disorders* (5th ed.; DSM-5; American Psychiatric Association [APA], 2013), a diagnosis of major depressive disorder (MDD) requires a person to meet several criteria during a two-week period, such as depressed mood throughout most of each day (which can also show up as irritability in teenagers), lack of interest in most activities, insomnia or sleeping too much, inability to concentrate, or recurring thoughts of death or suicidal ideation (APA, 2013). Individuals with MDD, which "frequently appears in puberty and is estimated to occur in at least one in 20 teenagers," struggle with maintaining relationships, attending work, or participating in school activities (Richmond, 2019, pp. 59–60). Depression rates in adolescents are high, with those aged 12–17 years old having a rate of 14.4 percent reported for major depressive episodes; teens also have the lowest rates of treatment (41.4 percent), according to the National Institute of Mental Health (NIMH) (2020).

In many young adult novels, authors give what might be called "red flags" to clue readers in to characters' intentions or motivations through dialogue, descriptions, or plot development. Teachers can guide adolescents as they navigate through novels in which characters display emotions and behaviors that might be related to depression. Educators may not be experts in mental health; however, they are often familiar with typical adolescent behaviors. Their expertise in working with literature specifically written for adolescents offers teachers the opportunity to engage teenage readers in an in-depth analysis and dialogue about characters who might be experiencing mental health issues or illnesses.

One book that lends itself to examining depression is *When Reason Breaks*, a young adult novel by Cindy L. Rodriguez (2015), which focuses on two protagonists who each live with symptoms of depression. The focus of this chapter centers on the two main mental health themes (depression and suicide) in *When Reason Breaks*, guiding readers through activities designed to help them navigate biases and preconceived notions while analyzing characters' emotions and behaviors. The novel provides a platform for readers to grapple with assumptions about depression and suicide and facts about mental illness as they take on the literacy focus of character analysis and study.

UNDERSTANDING DEPRESSION AND SUICIDE

As of 2017, more than 3 million adolescents aged 12–17 had at least one major depressive episode (NIMH, 2020). Major depression can occur along with anxiety and other mental disorders, and experts report that those with both anxiety and depression have more difficulty with recovery and are at higher risk for suicide (Cameron, 2007). In terms of suicide, research shows depression as a main predictor of suicidal thoughts; Cash and Bridge (2009) note, "20% [of those diagnosed with depression] will make more than one [suicide attempt]" during their adolescent years (p. 615). Rates of adolescent suicide have been on the rise in the past decade; Curtin (2020) reports that after "a period of stability from 2000 to 2007" suicide rates among youth ages 10–24 in the United States rose by 57.4 percent in 2018 (p. 3). High school teachers and families should pay attention to students' behaviors and provide resources for those who might be struggling with depression. Additionally, teachers should note that, according to recent research, "Depression is a disease that straddles all genders, ethnicities, races, and walks of life" and affects approximately 10 million Americans each year (Bailey et al., 2019, p. 603).

WHEN REASON BREAKS BY CINDY L. RODRIGUEZ

When Reason Breaks is a young adult novel by teacher and author Cindy L. Rodriguez, a U.S.-born Latina of Puerto Rican and Brazilian descent. The novel introduces readers to two young women, Emily Delgado, and Emily Davis, who goes by Elizabeth (her middle name) to reduce confusion when both girls are in English class with their teacher, Ms. Emelia Diaz. All three characters share the initials of Emily Dickinson, whose poetry acts as a thread throughout the narrative.

Both Emily and Elizabeth live with symptoms of depression, and the novel's chapters alternate between their perspectives. Rodriguez's (2015) novel starts in March when one of the two girls leaves an anonymous note for Ms. Diaz that reads, "Everything was all screwed up and it was my fault. The only way to clean up the mess was for me to disappear. And how else can that happen?" (p. 3). Her planned suicide involves taking an overdose of pills. The teacher discovers the letter and which of the teenagers wrote it; however, readers do not know until the book's last few chapters whether it is Emily or Elizabeth who penned the suicide note. Rodriguez disentangles this mystery for readers in an eight-month period, sharing details about the girls' personal, social, and academic lives, their various friendships and relationships, and their symptoms of depression.

GUIDING STUDENTS INTO THE TEXT

Mental Health Literacy

Throughout *When Reason Breaks*, Rodriguez shares the thoughts and feelings of Emily Delgado and Elizabeth Davis. By considering both young women's emotions and thoughts, readers can gain a better understanding of how their social-emotional experiences are connected to their actions and their relationships with family, friends, and others. To help readers reflect on Emily and Elizabeth's experiences, teachers can provide the following background terminology that is central to a mental health framework in Rodriguez's novel:

- *Depression:* In a period lasting more than two weeks, an individual has a depressed or dejected mood (chapters 10, 18, author's note), loss of interest or pleasure in everyday activities (chapter 16), and/ or symptoms such as *insomnia* (chapters 2, 5, 17, 18, 22, 27), *hypersomnia* (chapters 5, 23), *irritability* (chapters 15, 18, 19, 20, 38), and *lowered self-worth* (chapter 16, 27, 33) (APA, 2013).
- *Pills:* Medication (e.g., antianxiety, antidepressant, or sleeping pills) given for specific physical or psychological conditions (chapters 1, 2, 4, 5, 18, 23, 28, 34, 38, 41).
- *Suicidal ideation/suicidal:* A range of thoughts about death and suicide; thinking about one's own death (chapters 19, 23) (Harmer et al., 2020).
- *Suicide:* The intentional (as opposed to accidental) act of ending one's life (chapters 6, 23, 34, 36, 39, author's note).
- *Therapy and therapeutic techniques:* Meeting with a professional therapist, counselor, or doctor to identify, process, and manage mental health issues (chapters 23, 38, 40).

This list of mental health terms is provided to help readers understand Emily's and Elizabeth's experiences as the novel progresses. Teachers who review these terms with student readers can help them notice when these experiences occur for either character and whether the experiences occur independent of one another or in relation to each other.

Viewing Videos to Understand Characters

One option to help students better understand the author's perspective involves viewing videos by or about the author before reading the novel. For example, Cindy L. Rodriguez created an official book trailer video for *When Reason Breaks* (https://www.youtube.

com/watch?v=IFJzZCSP6vw), which introduces readers to the main characters, the setting, and the plot in an enticing visual format. This representation affords readers a way of "thinking about meaning in which language and visual text work in concert, and in which language is not the primary source through which meaning is mediated and represented" (Albers, 2014, p. 87).

In the case of *When Reason Breaks*, the video helps readers distinguish between Emily Delgado and Emily (Elizabeth) Davis, develop an understanding of the context (a suburban high school), and imagine the potential struggles within the novel. As students watch the video, they can be asked to consider their preconceived notions or biases about the characters of Emily and Elizabeth: What do they have in common and how are they different? What is the setting? How are the characters' personalities depicted through their appearances? How is information given through visual representations? Teachers can invite students to reflect on what insight the visual depictions of the characters might bring to their understanding of Elizabeth and Emily. Students can also predict how the characters might interact in and out of school and consider any foreshadowing of character development for Elizabeth, Emily, Ms. Diaz, and other characters in *When Reason Breaks*. Analysis of the video can also help students infer elements of plot development and conflicts in the novel.

List-Group-Label Reading Strategy

Before students read *When Reason Breaks*, teachers can tap into their students' prior knowledge about the subjects of depression and suicide through an adaptation of a *list-group-label* pre-reading strategy developed by Taba (1967). In adapting Taba's strategy, Boling and Evans (2008) asked students to create a communal list on a whiteboard of vocabulary words associated with a concept. Students were then guided through grouping words, using "common elements of the words and phrases to form groups" based on "parts of speech, similar meanings, types of characters, and so forth" (Boling & Evans, 2008, p. 61). Subsequently, students created a label connecting the words and relationships; the label, then, became a link used to form connections and prepare students to acquire new information (Boling & Evans, 2008).

By employing the *list-group-label* technique, teachers can lead readers through the creation of a visual representation of language and concepts in the novel, which may also benefit students with exceptionalities (including second language learners) who might require scaffolding of concepts while learning new vocabulary associated with a narrative.

In the case of *When Reason Breaks*, the concepts are "depression" and "suicide," and students can be asked to generate terms associated with those concepts based on their lived experiences and/or exposure to the terms in different contexts. For example, students might first individually write down terms that come to mind when they hear the words *depression* and *suicide* and be asked, before sharing with the group, to reflect on positive or negative connotations associated with the words. As this activity gives attention to matters of mental health, specifically that of depression and suicide, teachers can invite the school's mental health specialist to assist in facilitating classroom discussion and differentiating between terms that are culturally stigmatized as students share their terms with the group. Students' attention should also be drawn to how mental health terminology is not positive or negative but descriptive of behaviors. Teachers should be vigilant in asking students to frame their language in descriptive ways as to not contribute to the perpetuation of stigma associated with biases and stereotypes about mental illness.

This activity helps teachers tap into their students' understanding of the concepts of depression and suicide, recognize where students' lived experiences might intersect with the novel's content, aid students in identifying important mental health terms, and unpack their understandings and/or misconceptions of depression and suicide. After completing the *list-group-label* exercise, students are expected to approach the analysis of Emily's and Elizabeth's behaviors without having preconceived notions or biases influence their developing understandings of the characters.

GUIDING STUDENTS THROUGH THE TEXT

Character Analysis through Comparing and Contrasting

Just as readers have considered how Emily and Elizabeth might be portrayed as similar or different in Rodriguez's video trailer for

When Reason Breaks, students can continue to analyze the characters throughout their reading of the novel, looping back to consider whether their predictions about Emily and Elizabeth are confirmed or challenged as the plot unfolds. One compelling aspect of Rodriguez's novel is the cultural nuance embedded into the character development. Elizabeth Davis is a white cisgender female character identified in the book's front inside cover flap as a "Goth girl with an attitude problem." Elizabeth experiences a series of negative life events that puts her at heightened risk for depression: She has recently divorced parents (and is the one who discovers her father's infidelity), comes from a lower-income home with a single working mother, uses her artistic talents in somewhat provocative expressions, is externally emotionally reactive, and has a small group of friends. This characterization of Elizabeth is stereotypical and permits students to become more aware of how her behaviors might be dismissed at first as merely attributes of a Goth girl with an attitude problem. It also sets the stage for teen readers to become cognizant of misconceptions and assumptions they may make about how depression is manifested in fictional characters.

The other main character, Emily Delgado, is a Latina cisgender female character who is labeled in the book flap as "a smart, sweet girl, with a seemingly happy life" who "feels her depression closing in around her." Unlike Elizabeth, she does not present as a textbook case of someone with depression or an increased risk of suicidality. She comes from an upper-middle-class, intact family that seems respected by the community. Emily is popular, has a boyfriend, and excels in academics. Thus, she can fly under the radar and perhaps avoid being labeled as someone who is depressed or at risk for suicide. Additionally, Emily is not able to express her emotions, or for that matter, many aspects of herself, due to her father's very rigid standards.

Rodriguez paints an authentic picture of Emily's and Elizabeth's feelings, actions, interactions, and understandings of daily events. Students can examine the characters' navigation of their emotions, relationships, and behaviors while acknowledging the main characters' different cultural backgrounds. Students could also document the characters' shared symptoms of depression and potential risks for suicide by keeping track of the ways that Emily and Elizabeth behave and feel.

Teachers can employ a graphic organizer such as a Venn diagram or a T-chart through which students can track Emily's and Elizabeth's emotions, behaviors, relationships, and actions. If students are paired with partners, each pair could take responsibility for one of these aspects and share with the class during a whole-group discussion through a quick presentation or a virtually shared document. This activity could be enhanced a longer character analysis assignment in which students compare and/or contrast specific aspects of Elizabeth's or Emily's behaviors, social interactions, and physical and psychological well-being or depressive or suicidal thoughts in a written essay.

Literacy Quadrants

An additional strategy students can utilize while reading *When Reason Breaks* involves literacy quadrants, which is an instructional tool adapted from Frayer et al.'s (1969) model. Literacy quadrants "help students form concepts and learn new vocabulary by using four quadrants on a chart to define examples, non-examples, characteristics, and non-characteristics of a word" (Olan & Richmond, 2019, p. 90). Table 6.1 features an example of student prompts across four literacy quadrants.

Literacy quadrants can help readers focus on concepts and how they are related to others by using a sequence of interrogations about their experiences with a text: students can, in dialogue with a partner, engage in a series of procedures called "examine-predict-discuss" (Olan & Richmond, 2019, p. 91). Partners first examine their interpretations of depression, drawn from media portrayals, depictions in *When Reason Breaks*, and their assumptions about Emily's and Elizabeth's behaviors.

Table 6.1. Sample Literacy Quadrants with Student Prompts

Write terms or phrases that demonstrate how depression is depicted in the media (e.g., books, television, movies, etc.).	Write how these two characters with mental illness are portrayed in *When Reason Breaks* as compared to depictions of depression in the media. How are the characteristics similar or different?
List known media that depict characters with depression (reference the quadrant above).	Write to share your concerns, misconceptions, and challenges in understanding depression when reading *When Reason Breaks*.

Next, students take turns sharing their understandings and interpretations, predicting what they believe their partner's response indicates
about their comprehension and/or beliefs about depression. Finally,
partners read each other's literacy quadrants and revisit the novel,
discussing similarities or differences in their interpretations or assumptions; it is through this dialogic interaction that meaning making occurs.

Some interactions that evolve during this process include questioning
of shared experiences, comparing/contrasting ideas and examples, seeking approval of representations, checking for understanding, making
philosophical points related to depression in *When Reason Breaks*, and
discussing other texts with connections to similar themes. For this reason, teachers should invite the school's mental health specialist to join
them in facilitating the activity and discussion that ensues as a result of
student lists and responses.

For instance, a student might focus on Elizabeth's character, who
tells Ms. Diaz that she is "crazy" and "sick" because she feels like she
is not in control (p. 232). She also draws images in response to Ms.
Diaz's assignment about Emily Dickinson's poems: her drawings feature
bloody daggers and a person being isolated/imprisoned, and a lifeless
girl with a "straight-edged razor" lying in a pool of blood (p. 54, p. 132).
These drawings lead Ms. Diaz to be deeply concerned about Elizabeth
and to refer her to the school counselor, Ms. Gilbert. Students might
discuss how Elizabeth's behaviors and drawings fit with what they have
shared in their literacy quadrants about depression and whether their
representations align with known risks of depression and/or suicide.

Likewise, in considering Emily's character, teachers might point out
that Emily shares only a censored version of herself with her family, her
friends, and her boyfriend, among others. For example, in chapter 16,
when her friends Abby and Sarah hunt her down in the library because
Emily doesn't show up for lunch, they confront her about her avoidance,
noting that she has been isolating herself by missing mall trips, parties,
and movies. In response to their queries, Emily deflects and claims she
has "schoolwork and things at home" and is "tired" (p. 105). In chapter
28, during another discussion with her friends, Emily again relies on
defensive mechanisms of avoidance (not spending time with them) and
deflection (saying that her father's run for the legislature is interfering
with her free time). Moreover, in chapter 29, students could take note

of Emily's discussion with her friend Sarah, during which Emily says the days blend together and she feels "out of sync and almost entirely disconnected" from their friend Abby. Emily states, "It's not you. Nothing horrible has happened to me. . . . I don't know. Everything's all messed up, and maybe it's all my fault" (pp. 207–8). Later, Emily deletes her social media accounts and blocks her friends, including her boyfriend Kevin, on her phone. She also says she is exhausted, has "memory problems," and feels weak, irritable, and depressed. Students could interrogate their literacy quadrants to determine if their responses depict any similar emotions or behaviors. This characterization, deftly crafted by Rodriguez, exemplifies how Emily's self-invalidation depicts the ways in which depression is manifested in the text.

In conjunction with the school's mental health specialist, teachers might, at this point, want to share with students a list of "warning signs" of suicide such as those as shared by the National Association of School Psychologists (2020):

- suicide notes;
- direct statements or indirect comments about wanting to die;
- previous suicide attempts;
- symptoms of depression such as helplessness or hopelessness;
- risk-taking behaviors such as aggressive acts, playing with guns, or alcohol/substance abuse;
- saying goodbye to friends, giving away important items, or deleting posts or pictures online;
- self-injury such as cutting or scratching one's body;
- sudden changes such as acting up in class or skipping school or talking about having trouble concentrating; and/or
- showing an increased interest in weapons or hinting at a plan for suicide.

By providing this list, teachers, in collaboration with the school's mental health specialist, can further probe into students' understandings of suicide and depression and, perhaps, facilitate students' differentiating between the list of symptoms of depression and the list of potential warning signs that depression may have developed into thoughts of suicide. Through the literacy quadrants activity and guided dialogue, students and teachers can enhance their understanding of Rodriguez's portrayal of suicidal ideations through character development.

Moreover, from this activity, students can further revisit their assumptions about each character while simultaneously examining what the text tells readers about the characters. The outcome of this consideration is the revealing of discrepancies or variances between what teen readers notice about Emily's and Elizabeth's behaviors and what the author provides in terms of evidence about characters who live with depression and/or have suicidal ideations. For instance, when reading the character's anonymous "My Letter to the World" written with Ms. Diaz as the intended audience, students might focus on chapters 18 and 23 in which the character (which we identify as Emily unbeknownst to readers until chapter 34) discloses specific information about her attempts to seek help for insomnia, nightmares, and depression. In chapter 18, Emily describes vividly her nightmares and inability to sleep. She writes, "I knew then something deep down inside me was broken. It was the tiniest of cracks, like a pebble hitting a windshield on a highway—plink. No big deal, right? Wait a while. The crack will deepen and spread and permanently damage the once-strong glass" (p. 122). Emily knows at this point that she has to do something because she needed to sleep, so she goes to her mother because she was "desperate" and "hopeful, maybe, that she would be like other moms for once" and "listen and care" (p. 123); however, her mother's response is to open a bottle of pills and hand one to Emily with the instructions to take only half a pill. This action confirms Emily's assumption that her mother wasn't the person to offer her meaningful support in any way. Similarly, in chapter 28, Abby and Sarah dismiss Emily's disclosure about shutting her friends out; they tell Emily, "Snap out of it or take a pill or something and come out with us once in a while" (p. 200). In doing so, her friends have eliminated Emily's only remaining natural supports (those individuals not assigned to a prescribed role in her life such as teachers, therapists, doctors, etc.).

Likewise, in chapter 23, Emily goes to the doctor because her parents are concerned about her symptoms of aching all over and being tired. She is prescribed an antidepressant, and her mother is given a list of therapists to call; however, Emily chooses not to take the pills but, instead, rubs them like a worry stone and is concerned about the pills' side effects. She acknowledges that she wants to talk to "someone—not a shrink—but maybe you [Ms. Diaz]—about all of this," but she cannot because she is afraid that her teacher would have to "report it to someone else" (p. 162).

Through these chapters, Emily realizes she cannot depend on her parents because they are emotionally unavailable or unwilling to offer support other than pharmaceuticals. Emily acknowledges that if she shares her problems with Ms. Diaz, the teacher might suffer repercussions because of her status as a mandated reporter. Emily doesn't prioritize her own need for help with depression and suicidal ideation but, instead, seems to want to protect Ms. Diaz, which is not her role as a student. If students are exhibiting concerning behaviors or are aligning with characters' feelings about the adults, they can be reminded to work with empathetic adults who can provide safe options for help. Teachers might take this opportunity to point out Ms. Diaz's pattern of behavior as supportive to students who express emotional difficulties, for example, as she did when she spoke to Elizabeth when the student shared her drawings in chapter 10.

Through the responses and discussions associated with the metacognitive reflections, dialogues, and literacy quadrants activity, teachers can lead students toward a larger conversation about mental health issues connected with *When Reason Breaks*. Moreover, in using literacy quadrants, educators genuinely invite students to connect meaningfully to issues of depression, taking into account their prior knowledge of and experiences with mental health issues. Acknowledging Emily's and Elizabeth's experiences and emotions can help readers connect more fully with their perspectives as narrators in this novel.

Letters of Recommendation from Ms. Diaz

Often high school juniors and seniors are engaged in the process of applying for their first after-school job and/or gathering materials to submit with college applications. Letters of recommendation from their teachers are frequently sought as part of these processes. As part of writing letters of recommendation, educators emphasize strengths, skills, and leadership abilities as well as potential areas of growth. Additionally, they reflect on the student's character traits, behaviors, and academic contributions.

In this activity, students are asked to work independently to take the perspective of Ms. Diaz, the English teacher in *When Reason Breaks* while responding to the following prompt:

- Write a letter of recommendation from Ms. Diaz's perspective for Emily or Elizabeth for an after-school job or scholarship to college. What would their teacher say about each of the young women in terms of her academic strengths? What might be highlighted in terms of Emily or Elizabeth's personal strengths? What might Ms. Diaz note as areas for growth for each student?

Perspective taking is beneficial because it allows readers to move beyond the events in the narrative that they might associate with first impressions of depression or suicidal ideation in *When Reason Breaks.* Researchers in psychology have identified many benefits related to social perspective taking, which can be defined as "the ability to infer and understand another's viewpoint" (Gilman et al., 2014, p. 948). Benefits include the ability to build "positive interpersonal relationships" and "guide future personal, educational, and career choices" (Gilman et al., 2014, p. 948). For readers of Rodriguez's novel, the tendency might be to take up Emily's or Elizabeth's perspective; however, by taking up Ms. Diaz's perspective, readers may be able to acknowledge character traits of Emily and Elizabeth that they might not see at first when reading through their perspectives as narrators of the story. Moreover, Ms. Diaz—who, readers learn in the first pages, discovers a letter from one of the two girls and "drops everything, and runs as fast as her legs and heart allow" to find the student who has left the suicide note (p. 4)—is a character whose perspective changes throughout the novel. The note could have skewed her point of view about the person who left it for her; however, because Ms. Diaz has interacted with both young women, she was able to recognize and distinguish between Emily's and Elizabeth's characters.

Taking Ms. Diaz's perspective creates another layer for readers to examine characters' depression through the eyes of hope and perseverance rather than limitation and fear. By inviting students to write a letter of recommendation for a job or college application from Ms. Diaz's perspective, students can consider how taking a reflective stance facilitates deepening understanding of character portrayal and development in *When Reason Breaks.*

Discussion Questions

The purpose of the following discussion questions is to help readers continue to reflect and consider various perspectives on character development in general and on how depression is depicted through Emily's and Elizabeth's experiences in particular. As students progress through the text, there are many places that provide space to pause and ponder, reflect, and critically consider behaviors associated with mental illness and suicidal ideation displayed within character development. The following are some suggested questions that could serve as discussion or journal prompts:

- In chapter 1 (pp. 3–4), an unnamed girl is attempting suicide. What can you tell about her based on the details in the chapter? How do these actions depict behaviors associated with depression?
- Emily is hiding out at school reading a book when Elizabeth happens upon her in her hiding spot and asks her if she's okay (p. 108). What is Emily hiding, and how does Elizabeth know that?
- In the following passage, what does Elizabeth believe she knows about Emily, and how does that knowledge inform readers' perceived notions of each character? Why is Elizabeth grinning as she accuses Emily of lying? What might Elizabeth's motives be for confronting Emily in this way?

> With wide eyes, Emily asked, "Are you okay?"
> "I'm fine." Elizabeth smiled and sucked hard on her straw.
> "You're lying," she said with a grin. "Maybe, but this isn't about me. It's about you. Tell them. Get it over with, Delgado."
> Emily shook her head and hugged the book to her chest. "Tell them what?" (p. 110)

- Emily's depressive symptoms are mentioned throughout the story in a way where actions and behaviors depict brokenness, solitude, and darkness (pp. 67, 121, 287, 289). How does the author use specific word choice to convey Emily's emotions, fears, and development throughout the story?
- How do Emily's and Elizabeth's behaviors and interactions with family and friends reveal to readers their depressive states (pp. 54,

102, 131, 160, 193, 207, 268)? Which moments may have been opportunities for them to respond or intervene?

- In the novel, how does Rodriguez bring forth images of stereotypes
  about depression (pp. 67, 121, 200, 285)? Have stereotypes about
  individuals with depression changed since the book was published
  in 2015? Consider any research that might be available and/or reflect on how depression is portrayed in film, television, literature,
  and popular culture (e.g., songs, commercials, etc.).

- Refer to pp. 13, 19–22, 23–24. Our relationships with others, our
  background knowledge, and our cultural sensitivities can influence
  how we perceive and respond to what we read. Readers learn in
  chapter 3 that Elizabeth fought with her father the last time she
  saw him: "She remembered screams, fists, tears, and apologies. She
  remembered lying on the concrete in the fetal position, begging
  him to leave her alone" (p. 13). She also thought about "her sleep-
  less nights and about her mom—how she stares into space, how
  they can't have a real conversation. Her stomach clenched like it
  did every time her father called the house. Tommy was right. No
  one died, but something else did that day" (p. 13). In chapter 4,
  Emily's father is described as a successful lawyer involved in local
  politics; he and Emily speak in both Spanish and English. In chapter 5, readers learn that her mother "saw a bunch of specialists and
  had lots of tests done" and "swallowed a handful of pills every day"
  (p. 23). How might one's cultural background or personal experiences influence their response to Emily or Elizabeth as characters
  or how they are depicted? How might someone's cultural sensitivities influence how depression is described or treated?

- Refer to pp. 267–69. In chapter 38, Emily meets with the doctors
  in the hospital to discuss her progress. On day 4, she "starts to feel
  better physically, but she's angry and embarrassed" (p. 267). On day
  6, Emily feels "better overall" and doesn't want to "puke or throw
  something" when she sees her parents (p. 268). Rodriguez writes,
  "The monster inside her is weakened, but not dead"; the doctors
  ask her to make a "safety plan" and "sign a no-suicide contract,"
  but Emily "won't make any promises. This means more days in the
  hospital" (p. 269). Why do you think that Emily's feelings change

over a period of a week in the hospital? What is the "monster" that she describes? What changes might Emily go through after the first week of being in the hospital? Can you predict what will happen to Emily in the days to follow the scenes described earlier?

GUIDING STUDENTS OUT OF THE TEXT

A Call to Action

In *When Reason Breaks*, creative writing plays an important role in and out of Ms. Diaz's classroom. In her English classes, Ms. Diaz asks students to respond to Emily Dickinson's poetry through writing assignments and visual representations. Readers learn that Elizabeth is considered to be a talented artist, while Emily is called an "exceptional writer" (p. 125). Yet it is Elizabeth's poem that is published in the school newspaper albeit without her permission; this happens after Emily finds the poem in the classroom and gives it to Tommy (Elizabeth's boyfriend) to return to Elizabeth. Instead, Tommy turns the poem in to Kevin, who publishes the piece. Elizabeth's reaction to her poem being shared left her feeling exposed and vulnerable, and her response was anger and violence. She differentiates between the "personal" writing she does in her journal and writing for a public audience such as a newspaper (p. 119).

Responding to Poems in *When Reason Breaks*

Throughout *When Reason Breaks*, the character of Ms. Diaz provides students in her English classes, including Emily Delgado and Elizabeth Davis, with the opportunity to read and respond to poetry written by Emily Dickinson. Designed to help students experience the process of writing and responding to poetry like the characters do in the novel, the following activity facilitates students' responses to the character's creative expressions to further develop their understanding of Emily's and Elizabeth's feelings of depression in the novel.

Teachers can facilitate students' writing in response to one of Emily Dickinson's poems that Ms. Diaz teaches, or from one of the poems written by Emily Delgado or Elizabeth Davis in the novel. For example, in chapter 24, Elizabeth discusses with her English class a series of Emily Dickinson's stanzas (e.g., number 335, "Tis not that Dying hurts us so"; number 281, "Tis so appalling—it exhilarates"; and number 1062, "Caressed a Trigger absently"), focusing on Dickinson's "dark side" as a writer (p. 167). Students could choose one of these Dickinson poems as a springboard for their own writing, or instead, they could select Elizabeth Davis's poem (which starts "She holds the wishbone out to me" [p. 223]) or Emily Delgado's poetic response (in letter form) to Emily Dickinson's poem "The Soul has Bandaged moments" (p. 234). The goal of this activity is for the students to experience the process of writing in response to others' creative expressions and to build their understanding of the characters' feelings of depression throughout the book. These creative pieces, therefore, are not written with the intention to share publicly, though students might choose to share their poems.

In preparation for the final post-reading activity, teachers can invite students to debate the difference between writing for one's own purposes (to express ideas or get feelings out) and writing for a public audience (sharing ideas, emotions, information, or arguments). For example, students could explain, using textual evidence, why they believe Elizabeth felt violated in having her personal poem published by the school newspaper without her permission in chapter 31. Before the debate, students might make notes about how Emily Delgado, Elizabeth Davis, Tommy Bowles, or Kevin Wen-Massey use writing as a form of self-expression or not. Students might also jot down how they feel about sharing their own writing publicly.

Newspaper Articles and Public Service Announcements

A final activity for use with *When Reason Breaks* involves reading newspaper articles, which are often free and easily accessible to high school students. The assignment focuses on reading a variety of newspaper articles—either across time in one newspaper or across geographic areas in multiple newspapers during one specific time period, such as October, which is mental health awareness month. This activity provides students with a strategy for connecting the novel's focus (depression and suicide) with related current events or news reports.

For example, a regional newspaper such as the *Mining Journal* (published in Michigan's Upper Peninsula) featured several articles related to mental health in fall 2019. One article spotlighted a walk to raise funds and awareness for suicide prevention (Brown, 2019a). Another focused on a "LIVE Well" mental health campaign kick-off in a local community (Brown, 2019b). During the same time period, the *Detroit Free Press* featured the story of a 13-year-old Michigan native who became the face of Netflix's "Tell Them" campaign, a response to the popular video series *13 Reasons Why* about teen suicide, based in part on the young adult novel of the same name (Shamus, 2019). Students who read these articles could then create their own newspaper essay or public service announcement, synthesizing the information and relating it to high school audiences. Doing so can help students make connections between the novel and real-world journalism, which often blurs the lines between fiction and nonfiction. Moreover, this activity can help students make the connection that although Emily and Elizabeth are fictional characters they exhibit symptoms or warning signs that are common in individuals living with depression or have suicidal ideations, which they might recognize in a peer's behavior—or their own. Mental health awareness activities, such as a community walk for suicide prevention, provide a simple opportunity for people to jump ahead in stages of change because they are able to talk to someone and have a name and a face instead of cold calling an agency for support services.

Closing the Book

Both Elizabeth's struggles and Emily's experiences with depression, as well as Emily's attempted suicide, might cause readers to pause and reflect on their own struggles or experiences with depression or suicidal thoughts or ideations; however, *When Reason Breaks* closes on a positive note for both protagonists. Elizabeth makes a new start with her mother and younger sister Lily in chapter 37; they discuss a plan to be more open with one another, and Elizabeth gets a good night's rest for the first time in a year during a family slumber party. Emily, however, is at first resistant to participate in treatment for depression in the hospital in chapter 38. Moreover, she does not want to "create a safety plan and sign a no-suicide contract" (p. 269). She does begin to recognize her progress in chapter 40, stating that she begins to feel "stronger, lighter" (p. 275). Emily is "apprehensive" about leaving the "cozy sanctuary" of the hospital (p. 275). She knows from talks with her "shrinks" that she cannot control others' thoughts or actions; instead, she can only control "her own thoughts, actions, and emotions" (p. 276). Like many individuals who are actively recovering from depression, Emily feels uncertainty about her own future, yet she is willing to explore options with the support of family, friends, and mental health professionals.

As a final activity, teachers can have students identify strengths that Emily and Elizabeth exhibit as a method of unpacking and reflecting upon the hope that the two characters find toward the end of the novel. These strengths could include, for example, Emily's empathy for others and her use of writing to express her emotions, and Elizabeth's frankness and authenticity in her responses to others and willingness to take risks as she did with her interpretation of Dickinson's poem in chapter 8, with the line "words can wound" and a drawing of daggers dripping with blood (p. 54). Students can document Emily's and Elizabeth's strengths throughout the novel and consider how personal strengths can positively support people in their own journeys. Additionally, students could identify their own strengths and consider how those influence their behaviors, emotions, and actions.

CONCLUSION

The objective of this chapter has been to share ways to shepherd students through reading, analyzing, and responding to one book focused on characters living with depression and struggling with thoughts of suicide. By teaching *When Reason Breaks*, educators can provide students with intentional reading practices and activities designed to help them respond to the text and develop a better sense of mental health literacy. The activities suggested in this chapter aid readers in considering how young adults (living on the page, on the screen, or in the world around them) challenge assumptions about mental illness and open up conversations about depression and suicide as well as potential treatment options and resources for both issues. Educators are invited to help stop the stigma associated with mental illness and raise awareness of symptoms, behaviors, words, and actions related to depression and suicide by teaching a novel that can serve as a catalyst for students to interrogate their preconceived notions about depression and suicide while relating to characters who might be like them, or teens they know, in many ways.

REFERENCES

Albers, P. (2014). Visual discourse analysis. In P. Albers, T. Holbrook, & A. S. Flint (Eds.), *New methods of literacy research* (pp. 85–97). New York: Routledge. https://doi.org/10.4324/9780203104682

American Psychiatric Association. (2013). *Diagnostic and statistical manual of mental disorders* (5th ed.). Washington, DC: American Psychiatric Publishing. https://doi.org/10.1176/appi.books.9780890425596

Bailey, R. K., Mokonogho, J., & Kumar, A. (2019). Racial and ethnic differences in depression: Current perspectives. *Neuropsychiatric Disease and Treatment, 15*, 603–9. https://doi.org/10.2147/NDT.S128584

Boling, C. J., & Evans, W. H. (2008). Reading success in the secondary classroom. *Preventing School Failure, 52*(2), 59–66. https://doi.org/10.3200/PSFL.52.2.59-66

Brown, C. (2019a, September 4). Saturday walk to raise funds, awareness for suicide prevention. *Mining Journal.* https://www.miningjournal.net/news/front-page-news/2019/09/saturday-walk-to-raise-funds-awareness-for-suicide-prevention/

Brown, C. (2019b, September 1). LIVE well mental health campaign kicks off today. *Mining Journal.* https://www.miningjournal.net/news/front-page-news/2019/09/live-well-mental-health-campaign-kicks-off-today/

Cameron, O. G. (2007). Understanding comorbid anxiety and depression. *Psychiatric Times, 24*(4). http://www.psychiatrictimes.com/anxiety/understanding-comorbid-depression-and-anxiety

Cash, S. J., & Bridge, J. A. (2009). Epidemiology of youth suicide and suicidal behavior. *Current Opinion in Pediatrics, 21*(5), 613–19. https://doi.org/10.1097/MOP.0b013e32833063e1

Curtin, S. C. (2020). State suicide rates among adolescents and young adults aged 10–24: United States, 2000–2018. *National Vital Statistics Reports, 69*(11), 1–10. https://www.cdc.gov/nchs/data/nvsr/nvsr69/nvsr-69-11-508.pdf

Frayer, D., Frederick, W. C., & Klausmeier, H. J. (1969). *A schema for testing the level of cognitive mastery.* Madison: Wisconsin Center for Education Research.

Gilman, R., Rice, K. G., & Carboni, I. (2014). Perfectionism, perspective taking, and social connection in adolescents. *Psychology in the Schools, 51*(9), 947–59. https://doi.org/10.1002/pits.21793

Harmer, B., Lee, S., Duong, T. V. H., & Saadabadi, A. (2020, November 23). *Suicidal Ideation.* Treasure Island, FL: StatPearls Publishing.

National Association of School Psychologists. (2020). *Save a friend: Tips for teens to prevent suicide.* https://www.nasponline.org/resources-and-pub lications/resources-and-podcasts/school-climate-safety-and-crisis/mental -health-resources/preventing-youth-suicide/save-a-friend-tips-for-teens-to -prevent-suicide

National Institute of Mental Health. (2020). *Major depression.* https://www .nimh.nih.gov/health/statistics/major-depression.shtml

Olan, E. L., & Richmond, K. J. (2019). Using literacy quadrants in preparing teachers of writing: Reflective tools for identity, agency, and dialogue. *Teaching/Writing: Journal of Writing Teacher Education,* 6(1), article 6. https:// scholarworks.wmich.edu/wte/vol6/iss1/6

Richmond, K. J. (2019). *Mental illness in young adult literature: Exploring real struggles through fictional characters.* Santa Barbara, CA: ABC-CLIO: Libraries Unlimited.

Rodriguez, C. L. (2015). *When reason breaks.* New York: Bloomsbury.

Shamus, K. J. (2019, October 9). She was 13 when she first attempted suicide. *Detroit Free Press.* https://www.freep.com/story/news/local/michigan/2019/10/09/ teen-suicide-prevention-riley-juntti-13-reasons-why-netflix/3844718002/

Taba, H. (1967). *Teacher's handbook for elementary social studies.* Boston, MA: Addison-Wesley.

U.S. Department of Health and Human Services, National Institute of Mental Health. (2019). *Mental illness: Prevalence of any mental disorder among adolescents.* https://www.nimh.nih.gov/health/statistics/mental-illness .shtml#part_155771

7

"I'M NOT LIKE *THAT*"

Reading *Heroine* to Engage Students in Conversations and Research about Opioid Use Disorder

Amanda Rigell, Arianna Banack, and Allen Rigell

Contemporary young adult literature (YAL) and mainstream media are beginning to tell more stories about people who face mental health challenges, including a focus on substance use disorder. Stories about the psychological and emotional impact of substance use disorders (SUD) are especially important for adolescents to explore, as the United States faces a national opioid crisis (Department of Health and Human Services [HHS], 2019). Furthermore, student understandings of substance use disorders may be intertwined with stigma and misconceptions about how addiction begins. As teachers, we can expose our students to narratives about substance abuse, and scaffold students' research skills, to help them become more informed about our national health crisis.

Mindy McGinnis's (2019) young adult novel, *Heroine*, can help accomplish this goal as it demonstrates how opioid use disorder (OUD), a type of SUD, can evolve from a medical professional's legal prescription to an addiction that is difficult to relinquish on one's own. Using YAL in the classroom can help students understand and destigmatize mental illness (Richmond, 2019), an issue that *Heroine* addresses poignantly. This chapter aims to assist teachers in integrating the novel *Heroine* into their curriculum as a means of teaching critical research skills and contextualizing an understanding of addiction. The resources and strategies offered here are designed to strengthen students' ability to make real-world connections through research and intertextual connections.

UNDERSTANDING SUBSTANCE USE DISORDER

According to the Centers for Disease Control (CDC), significant percentages of American high schoolers misuse drugs and alcohol: by grade 12, two-thirds of students have tried alcohol; half have used marijuana; and nearly two in 10 have used prescription medication without a prescription (CDC, 2020). According to the National Institute on Drug Abuse (2020), "people are most likely to begin abusing drugs—including tobacco, alcohol, and illegal and prescription drugs—during adolescence and young adulthood" (para. 1). Illicit use of legally distributed substances like opioids is dangerous, not only because of its biochemical risks, such as respiratory depression, seizures, heart failure, and death, but also because adolescents who misuse prescription opioids are also significantly more likely to concurrently engage in behaviors like dangerous driving, violence, unsafe sexual choices, use of other drugs and alcohol, and suicide (Bhatia et al., 2020).

The community presence of opioids is so widespread that the Department of Health and Human Services recently declared a public health emergency connected to the use and abuse of both prescription and non-prescription opioids in the United States (2019). The Office of Juvenile Justice and Delinquency Prevention also recently declared that "more than 4,000 deaths among youth ages 15–24 were attributed to opioid overdose" (2020, para. 1). While the opioid epidemic continues to be a public health crisis, adolescent substance abuse is often left unaddressed in classrooms. This chapter aims to empower teachers to facilitate difficult conversations contextualized in a young adult novel that offers an unflinching look at the opioid epidemic.

HEROINE BY MINDY MCGINNIS

Heroine focuses on the story of high school senior and star softball catcher, Mickey Catalan, whose traumatic car accident results in intensive hip surgery and a prescription for OxyContin, an opioid that is often prescribed as a painkiller. With the softball team making a historic state championship run, Mickey wants nothing more than to resume her position as a catcher as soon as possible. She realizes she's able to push herself harder in rehabbing her hip and in softball practice when she has taken a few OxyContin. But when Mickey's prescription runs out and she realizes she depends on the pills to get through her days, she must find another way to get more OxyContin—and eventually heroin—while trying to preserve her identity as the perfect student-athlete, daughter, and role model to those around her.

With adolescent heroine Mickey Catalan driving the plot, McGinnis explores the trauma of a SUD and the road to recovery while challenging common stereotypes of people addicted to legal and illegal opioids. McGinnis shows how opioids can weave their way through a community and touch the lives of adolescents who appear to have it all together.

GUIDING STUDENTS INTO THE TEXT

Mental Health Literacy

Throughout *Heroine*, the protagonist and narrator, Mickey, describes not only her escalating opioid misuse but also intellectual and emotional justifications for her behavior. Her confiding tone creates an intimacy between character and reader that intensifies our realization that she is in grave danger as her use escalates. She begins misusing her own legally prescribed OxyContin, then illegally obtaining OxyContin, and eventually buying and using heroin. The book's stark moments depicting opioid use demand background knowledge and contextualization to support students' progression through the novel.

To build background knowledge and scaffold vocabulary acquisition, this chapter recommends nonfiction articles centered on the opioid crisis, along with a glossary of terminology relevant to Mickey's story that is aligned with the *Diagnostic and Statistical Manual of Mental Disorders* (5th ed.; DSM–5; American Psychiatric Association [APA], 2013). As students apply the noted vocabulary to Mickey's experience, they can be better prepared to understand Mickey's actions and emotions throughout the course of the novel. Although many of the indicators of OUD are present throughout the novel, we have listed particularly relevant chapters to help teachers provide guiding examples for their students.

- *Substance use disorder (SUD):* Symptoms that result from the use of a substance that someone continues to use even though it causes the individual problems. *Substance use disorder* is a general term that encompasses the misuse of substances including alcohol, prescription and illicit drugs, and tobacco; this general term is used in the DSM-5 rather than *addiction*. *Opioid use disorder* is a specific substance use disorder that has its own name and symptoms (APA, 2013).

- *Opioid use disorder (OUD):* A problematic pattern of opioid use leading to clinically significant impairment or distress, indicated in several ways, including the following:

  - Taking opioids in larger amounts or for a longer time than intended (chapters 7, 9, 19, 20)
  - Spending a significant amount of time obtaining opioids (chapters 20, 36)
  - Cravings or urges to take opioids (chapters 24, 39, 43, 44, 47)
  - Giving up participation in meaningful activities (chapters 37, 55)
  - Recurrent opioid use in situations in which it is hazardous (chapters 41, 43)
  - Recurrent use resulting in failure to fulfill work, school, or home obligations (chapters 35, 43, 46, 47)
  - Unsuccessful efforts to cut down or control use (chapters 25, 27)
  - Continuing to use opioids even when they cause interpersonal problems (chapters 16, 24, 26, 27, 29, 32)
  - Using opioids even when they are worsening one's physical or psychological health (chapters 13, 24, 34, 36)
  - Increased tolerance to opioids (chapters 6, 14, 16, 19, 21, 46, 47)
  - Withdrawal symptoms (chapters 7, 24, 52) (APA, 2013)

- *Harm reduction:* A set of practical strategies grounded in social justice and aimed at reducing negative consequences associated with drug use (National Harm Reduction Coalition, 2020), including providing information about safer drug use, clean supplies for drug use, psychosocial support, and overdose prevention and reversal (e.g., naloxone).

This glossary may be expanded and used as a supportive resource to build students' mental health vocabulary and comprehension throughout the novel study. Students can keep a physical or virtual copy of the glossary for themselves, and a class copy can be displayed in the classroom (virtually or physically) for everyone to access.

Establishing a Reflective Stance: Examining Preconceptions about Opioid Use Disorder

In addition to familiarizing themselves with the definitions of SUD and OUD, students and teachers may also examine their preconceived notions about these topics. To facilitate critical self-reflection, and as a way to introduce research and synthesis skills, students can prepare to research portrayals of opioid use in the media. Teachers can ask the school's media specialist to visit the classroom to help students understand how to find multiple credible sources and conduct effective internet searches using research questions. Teachers can either provide students with the following research questions or have students create their own questions with assistance from the media specialist and teacher: Where do we see substance use disorders represented in the media and advertising? How are substance use disorders, including opioid use disorder, represented in stories we hear, see, and share?

After finding media or advertising materials that portray SUD, students are encouraged to engage in a think-pair-share so they are exposed to their peer's research. Each pair should consider the follow: How do these portrayals influence our preconceived notions about substance use and substance use disorders? Do they challenge our perceptions or affirm them? What stereotypes might these resources be supporting or pushing against? Whose experiences are not represented in these resources? After discussion, each pair can share one of their media clips or advertisements with the class along with a synthesis of their discussion. This activity helps prepare students to engage in research and synthesis, which are foundational skills for the unit featured throughout this chapter.

Exploring Research: Author Interviews about *Heroine*

Young adult novel authors have long written about difficult subjects and experiences. The stark realities of OUD shared in *Heroine* can be difficult for some readers to navigate. Understanding why McGinnis chose to craft a narrative about a female athlete, why she chose to write about opioid and heroin use, and why her publisher fought to get the novel in line for release are all details that provide powerful context and perspective-taking opportunities for students. The interviews listed below offer a few options of short, engaging interviews that provide unique insights about the book and author. Most important, they ground the novel in the author's observations of and research on the impact of opioids in communities. Teachers can also work with students to conduct additional research in identifying interviews and articles that share information on the author and her work in preparing and writing the novel.

- "Author Interview: Mindy McGinnis." https://blog.libro.fm/author -interview-mindy-mcginnis/
- "Six Questions: An Interview with Mindy McGinnis, Author of *Heroine*." https://the nerddaily.com/ mindy-mcginnis-author-interview/
- "Q&A: Mindy McGinnis Author of *Be Not Far from Me*." https:// mikeschlossbergauthor/com/2019/05/09/six-questions-an-inter view-with-mindy-mcginnis-author-of-heroine/

Teachers can ask students to complete a jigsaw activity in small groups to share key takeaways from these interviews. Each group could read one interview and work together to identify three main points, two important quotes, and one question the interview prompted them to consider. Students can either create a poster or visual presentation with this information and then share with the class one by one, or groups can pair up and share with each other until each group has discussed all three interviews.

This activity gives students a chance to talk about why someone would write a book about the opioid epidemic, begins to ground students in research, and provides them practice with presenting information to their peers. Through this activity, students are presented with reliable nonfiction sources they can use as exemplars when they conduct their own research throughout the unit. By exposing students to multiple examples of credible sources, and asking them to synthesize and share their learning, students can prepare for the culminating research task shared at the conclusion of this chapter.

GUIDING STUDENTS THROUGH THE TEXT

Understanding the Opioid Epidemic through Synthesizing Nonfiction Texts

Table 7.1 shares three suggested nonfiction texts paired with specific chapters of the novel to help scaffold students' understanding of the opioid crisis in tandem with Mickey's developing addiction. As Mickey's addiction intensifies, students can continue to gain knowledge and synthesize their understanding of literary and informational texts about the opioid crisis. In the activities suggested here, students engage in synthesis of their understanding of each nonfiction article independently but will be asked to pull their learning together as a group just before the conclusion of the novel and after reading all of the identified nonfiction texts. As students read the articles, they can keep track of key facts and text-to-text connections on a graphic organizer (see table 7.1) as a means of synthesizing their newfound context and understanding about *Heroine* and opioid use disorder.

After reading chapter 5 of *Heroine*, students can view a video, "The Facts on America's Opioid Epidemic" (Al-Hlou et al., 2017), which provides a brief history of the opioid crisis from the 1990s to the present. Chapter 5 describes the days just after Mickey is prescribed OxyContin. The reader gets the sense that she is beginning to depend on it as Mickey states, "I couldn't even get a shower if it wasn't for the Oxy, and my teammates tossing the bottle around like a scuffed up softball sets me a little on edge" (p. 31). As an alternate option and activity following this chapter, teachers could have students read the article "Opioid History: From 'Wonder Drug' to Abuse Epidemic" (Moghe, 2016). Gathering factual information about the opioid epidemic is a key component in building the foundation for rich discussion and connection-making when reading *Heroine*, as well as preparing students to research the epidemic in more depth in the culminating task for this novel.

After reading chapter 28, students can listen to a Mayo Clinic Q&A podcast, "Opioid Crisis Worsens during COVID-19 Pandemic" (Gazelka, 2021) about the opioid crisis, which will facilitate text-to-text and text-to-world connections, as well as provide students with examples of reliable sources. While the entire podcast is useful, students can listen to minutes 1:55–7:08 if teachers do not have time to play the entire 27 minutes in class. This podcast provides students with definitions of OUD, discusses the stigma of addiction, and provides signs indicative of opioid use disorder. The podcast also discusses the repercussions of the opioid crisis on communities and families. This information can be helpful in facilitating a discussion about how there are many people who have experiences similar to what Mickey describes in the book.

After students have read chapter 40, teachers could direct them to view the interactive article titled "The Class of 2000 'Could Have Been Anything'" (Levin, 2019). The article focuses on a small town in Ohio, similar to the setting of *Heroine*, and features interactive pictures and stories students can explore independently or with small discussion groups. There are explicit connections to *Heroine*, as multiple interviewees describe how their addiction to OxyContin started with a car accident or other significant injury. The article's author and contributors made efforts to contact all 110 members of the town's graduating class for extensive interviews. Their conversations with 49 of the classmates reveal that more than 30 percent of them reported a former or current opioid addiction (Levin, 2019). As students read this article, they can use the graphic organizer shown in table 7.1 as a tool to consider how this article influences their understanding of the opioid crisis. Additionally, to explicitly connect the articles to the text, students can also use the graphic organizer to support connections from the nonfiction articles with textual evidence from *Heroine* and engage in synthesis of all their nonfiction sources.

Table 7.1. Graphic Organizer for Nonfiction Articles and *Heroine*

Title of Nonfiction Article	Three Key Notes from Article	Connections to *Heroine* *How does the article connect to Heroine? What similarities and differences exist between these stories and Mickey's story?*
"The Class of 2000 'Could Have Been Anything'" (Levin, 2019)	Scioto County in Ohio has the highest number of fatal drug overdoses and drug-related arrests.	The 2020 yearbook article said, "Melissa Pace was in high school chorus and a class officer. She was prescribed opioids after a car accident her senior year" (Levin, 2019), and right after Mickey gets released from the hospital after her accident, she says, "I couldn't get through a shower if it wasn't for the Oxy" (p. 31). So many people started with a prescription from their doctor to treat pain and ended with addiction.
"The Facts on America's Opioid Epidemic" (Al-Hlou et al., 2017)	The opioid epidemic kills about 90 Americans every day.	Throughout *Heroine* there were many obituaries featured that showcase opioid overdose, including three of Micky's friends: Josie, Derrick, and Luther.
Mayo Clinic Q&A podcast: "Opioid Crisis Worsens during COVID-19 Pandemic"	Opioid use disorder is defined as the overuse or uncontrolled use of an addictive substance.	Mickey would be able to be diagnosed with an "OUD" based on the discussion during the podcast because of the overuse of her prescription. She continues to obtain more pills from Edy after her prescription runs out.

Synthesis: *What new understandings about opioid use and abuse have you gained from reading our nonfiction texts? How have they influenced your understanding of Mickey und her friends in Heroine? Create a graphic, either hand drawn or using online tools, to represent your* learning from reading the research and connecting it to our novel. This graphic may take the form of a static drawing or an interactive website such as a Prezi. You will present your graphic to the class to share your synthesis.

All of these resources, and their corresponding activities, provide important context about the opioid epidemic, along with personal vignettes of substance misuse or stories of loved ones lost to addiction.

Making Connections: A Gallery Walk

To help scaffold students in developing their research skills, students can work in small groups to create stations for a gallery walk activity. Students might engage in this activity after reading chapter 28 of *Heroine* because it is at this point that students will have read three nonfiction texts and explored examples of reliable research. If students require additional scaffolding on how to locate and evaluate credible sources, teachers can work in collaboration with the school's media specialist to guide students through accessing and navigating the school or community library resources. Teachers can also find ways to infuse additional instruction and support in identifying, assessing, and examining bias within nonfiction sources.

As teachers begin this activity, direct students to locate short nonfiction articles, photographs, songs or song lyrics, interviews, or video clips to display at each station of the gallery walk. The identified resources should connect directly to either the history of the opioid epidemic, symptoms of opioid abuse, or harm-reduction tactics. Students can also prepare a bulleted list of key points presented within each selected resource. After students have identified their resources, they can share their ideas with the teacher to ensure that each source is reliable, that the information is factual, and that each group has selected materials unique to those selected by their peers.

After each group has solidified their resource selection and prepared their key points, they can rotate to the other groups' stations. Depending on the resources selected, students can spend at least 5–10 minutes at each station before rotating to the next station. At each station, students can complete a graphic organizer (see table 7.2) in which they document the title of the resource, the key points, and a connection to *Heroine*.

At the conclusion of the activity, the teacher can ask each group to share one fact they learned from another group and one connection they

Table 7.2. Making Connections Gallery Walk Example

Title of Resource	Key Points	Connection to Heroine
	What key points did the group prepare for you? Add two key points of your own.	*What text-to-text connections can you identify between this resource and the novel?*
Include title of resource here	Include key points here	Include text-to-text connections here

made to *Heroine*. Teachers can also pace this activity out over multiple days with the initial days dedicated to research and synthesis of the group's station and the remaining days spent participating in the gallery walk and learning from peers.

Peritextual Features, Mickey, and the Opioid Epidemic

In each chapter of *Heroine*, McGinnis embeds the peritextual feature of an epigraph, introducing the chapter with a single word and its definition. Teachers can leverage these epigraphs to facilitate check-in discussions at regular intervals throughout the novel. Teachers can use the following guiding questions to encourage partner conversations, small-group discussions, or brief warm-up discussions:

- Why do you think McGinnis chose this word as the epigraph for the chapter?
- What word would you choose as the reader and why?
- Which of the informational texts you have examined does this word bring to mind and why?

Students may also choose to investigate each word further, especially those directly related to substance abuse seen in the following chapters:

- Chapter 4: *family*
- Chapter 14: *tolerance*
- Chapter 15: *addict*
- Chapter 24: *withdrawal*
- Chapter 38: *heroin*

Students can discuss if the provided epigraph aligns with their research of SUDs and how the epigraph enhances the reader's understanding of each chapter. As the definitions provided in the book are brief, students can practice their research skills by providing additional detail to each epigraph and discussing as a whole class what additional information needs to be added to understand selected terms.

Discussion Questions

Fishbowl Discussion: Analyzing Opiod Use Disorder and Supporting Characters

Conversations about OUD must consider the impact of opioid use on entire communities. Using *Heroine* as a lens for discussion, students can examine the community-level effects of opioids through conversation surrounding the supporting characters. Teachers may consider a fishbowl activity, or an approach to engaging in a Socratic seminar conversation, to discuss the following text-based questions centered on supporting characters. Students can prepare responses to the following questions in the previous class, or they can answer them on the day of the discussion, depending on allotted class time. The teacher can print the questions on small strips of paper and place them in any container. About four or five students sit in an inner circle in the center of the classroom, and the remaining students sit in an outer circle, facing the small group at the center of the room. Students seated within the inner circle begin by extracting a question from the container and engaging with one another in peer-to-peer discussion of the selected question. When students feel they have sufficiently answered the question, they can select another question from the container. Each group can spend a predetermined amount of time in the center of the circle before moving to the outer circle and providing an opportunity for a new group to rotate to the inner circle. Teachers may also encourage students to "tap" each other out of the inner circle until all students have been given a chance to participate in the conversation. Teachers can reference the following questions for this discussion:

- How does Mickey try to hide her substance abuse from her friends and loved ones? Why do you believe these are successful for so long? (chapters 24, 34, 35, 36)
- How does Mickey rationalize her substance abuse? How do these rationalizations change throughout the novel? (chapters 7, 10, 13, 21, 45)
- How do Luther and Josie challenge our perception of the words *addict* or *junkie*? (chapters 23, 34, 45)
- How would you describe Devra's role in Mickey's life? (chapters 29, 52, 53, 54)
- What aspects of Mickey's friendship with Carolina impact, or are impacted by, Mickey's opioid use? (chapters 17, 20, 24, 34, 36, 54)

GUIDING STUDENTS OUT OF THE TEXT

A Call to Action

Research in Action

The Society for Public Health Education (Hampton et al., 2019) asserted that public health education is the key to preventing opioid addiction and advocates "building opioid misuse prevention education into school curricula" (p. 15) as a primary intervention in preventing SUDs and helping heal communities. To bring the novel study to a close, students can collectively create an interactive infographic about OUDs using the research skills and findings they have documented throughout their reading of the novel.

The infographic is intended to function as an authentic, standards-based task for students, as well as an upstream educational resource for the classroom, school, or wider community. Students may contribute individually to the infographic or work in small groups depending on teacher preference and class size.

Teachers may wish to consider themselves the "editor in chief" of the infographic created by students—that is, students can submit their contributions to their teacher to compile. An example is included in figure 7.1.

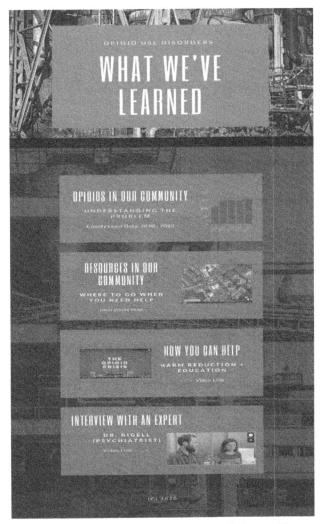

Figure 7.1. Example of Interactive Infographic on Opioid Use Disorder

The interactive infographic may be constructed in a modular format, with each student or group of students creating a module. Students can research and report information specific to their community, including the following:

- Research on the support services their school or community offers for substance use disorders

- Research definitions of OUD that people in the community need to know (students may revisit the glossary they developed during pre-reading as a resource)
- Research about drugs prevalent in their community and the history of those drugs in the community
- Research about how community members can support people struggling with SUDs and research conducted via interviews with school counselors or community mental health providers
- Research from multiple perspectives about community substance use interventions (e.g., law enforcement, mental health care providers, health departments, city- and county-level social services offices)
- Research healing work that organizations are already undertaking. As a starting point, the following resources illustrate research and active interventions that scientists, health care providers, and community members are trying and evaluating as they attempt to facilitate recovery and healing:

  ◦ "HEALing Communities Across America," a research spotlight describing community-specific research by the National Institutes of Health (2020)
  ◦ "East Tennessee County Teaching Kids How to Use Narcan," a profile of a harm reduction strategy and its proponents in rural Tennessee (Gallant, 2020).

Once students have created and submitted their modules, students can work in groups to compile them into an infographic. The infographic may be presented at a schoolwide event or a community gathering, or it may be distributed digitally to students, parents, and community stakeholders.

Many online infographic creators have a sharing option that allows users to create hyperlinks. This functionality means that each module of the infographic may link viewers to a discrete resource contributed by students. For example, a report in layman's terms about county-wide statistics related to opioid use; an interactive Google Map, Google Tour, or Google Earth project locating and explaining local treatment and recovery centers; or video interviews with local mental health, public health, or harm reduction leaders. In other words, the infographic is designed to function as a customized community tool for education about OUDs and recovery.

This student-created resource may be distributed digitally through school newspapers, school websites, school social media accounts, school e-mails or text messages, or via school-parent communication apps. Presentation and distribution of the infographic as a community resource offers authenticity to this culminating task and connects the novel study with valuable English language arts research skills.

Closing the Book

"Chalk" Talk Reflection

Following the conclusion of the novel, students can work in groups to complete a written dialogue in which they share their thoughts about the novel's impact on their perceptions of opioid use and reply to one another in a structured, collaborative format (e.g., writing on poster paper, Padlets, Google JamBoard, etc.). Students can answer the following questions as they reflect on their learning throughout the unit:

- How do Mickey's experiences connect with those we've encountered in our nonfiction articles?
- On page 69, Mickey says, "I'm not like that." How does her denial of her OUD influence her recovery? How does it influence her relationships?
- In what ways has the novel, and your research throughout, impacted the way you think about addiction and opioid use?
- Which was more influential on your perceptions: the nonfiction articles or the novel? Why?
- How can we be critical of the portrayals of opioid use we see in texts, media, and advertising? What have we learned that we can apply to media representation?

This shared space can be used to collectively assess the significant takeaways from the novel study and provides a moment to consider how each student hopes to move forward in their understanding of opioid and other substance use disorders. Reflecting in real time and seeing their peers' reflections is a dynamic way to conclude the novel. Furthermore, a wrap-up conversation grounded in what students have learned allows them to reflect on the engagingly educative power of narrative and how they incorporated narrative into their research project about the opioid epidemic.

CONCLUSION

Heroine's unflinching exploration of the arc of SUD, intervention, and steps toward recovery can be challenging content for readers of any age. While it is a work of fiction, *Heroine* tackles a heartbreaking reality of our time. The resources, discussion tools, and culminating activities presented throughout this chapter are designed to help teachers and students navigate the difficult topic of OUD through the proactive acts of reflection and research. Empowering students with research literacies gives them tools to sort fact from fiction when they face complicated conversations about mental health. Discussion, education, and intervention grounded in research are essential components of mental health literacy, within and beyond the classroom.

REFERENCES

Al-Hlou, Y., Katz, J., & Jordan, D. (2017, October 26). The facts on America's opioid epidemic. *New York Times.* https://www.nytimes.com/video/health/policy/100000005515818/the-opioid-epidemic-what-you-need-to-know.html

American Psychiatric Association. (2013). *Diagnostic and statistical manual of mental disorders* (5th ed.). Washington, DC: American Psychiatric Publishing. https://doi.org/10.1176/appi.books.9780890425596

Bhatia, D., Mikulich-Gilbertson, S. K., & Sakai, J. T. (2020). Prescription opioid misuse and risky adolescent behavior. *Pediatrics, 145*(2), e20192470. https://doi.org/10.1542/peds.2019-2470

Centers for Disease Control. (2020). *Teen substance use and risks.* https://www.cdc.gov/ncbddd/fasd/features/teen-substance-use.html

Department of Health and Human Services. (2019). *What is the U.S. opioid epidemic?* https://www.hhs.gov/opioids/about-the-epidemic/index.html

Gallant, K. (2020). *East Tennessee county teaching kids how to use Narcan.* WKRN.com. https://www.wkrn.com/news/east-tennessee-county-teaching-kids-how-to-use-narcan/

Gazelka, H. (Host) (2021, January 1). Opioid crisis worsens during COVID-19 pandemic [Audio podcast episode]. In Mayo Clinic Q & A. Mayo Clinic. https://newsnetwork.mayoclinic.org/discussion/mayo-clinic-qa-podcast-opioid-crisis-worsens-during-covid-19-pandemic/

Hampton, C., Buckley, J., Auld, M. E., & Drewiske, K. (2019). *A nation in crisis: A health education approach to preventing opioid addiction.* (Policy brief). Washington, DC: Society for Public Health Education.

Levin, D. (2019). The class of 2000 "Could have been anything." *New York Times.* https://www.nytimes.com/interactive/2019/12/02/us/opioid-crisis-high-school-teenagers.html

McGinnis, M. (2019). *Heroine.* New York: Katherine Tegen Books.

Mogue, S. (2016, May 12). *Opioid history: From "wonder drug" to abuse epidemic.* CNN Health. https://www.cnn.com/2016/05/12/health/opioid-addiction-history/index.html

National Harm Reduction Coalition. (2020). *Principles of harm reduction.* https://harmreduction.org/about-us/principles-of-harm-reduction/

National Institute on Drug Abuse. (2020, June 2). *Introduction.* https://www.drugabuse.gov/publications/principles-adolescent-substance-use-disorder-treatment-research-based-guide/introduction

National Institutes of Health. (2020). *HEALing communities across America.* https://heal.nih.gov/news/stories/HEALing-Communities

Office of Juvenile Justice and Delinquency Prevention. (2020). *Supporting youth and families impacted by opioid use.* https://ojjdp.ojp.gov/programs/opioid-abuse?utm_source=ncjrs.gov&utm_medium=web&utm_campaign=ncjhomepagecontent

Richmond, K. J. (2019). *Mental illness in young adult literature: Exploring real struggles through fictional characters.* Santa Barbara, CA: ABC-CLIO / Libraries Unlimited.

READING A HERO'S JOURNEY THROUGH *OCDANIEL*

Caitlin Corrieri and Elyana Genovese

Obsessive-compulsive disorder (OCD) is diagnosed in approximately one in 200 youth, with research suggesting that in a large high school the disorder may be present in about 20 adolescents (Wagner, 2009). OCD features repetitive thinking and behaviors (American Psychiatric Association [APA], 2013), each of which are key criteria in identifying obsessive-compulsive disorder. Specifically, OCD is characterized by the occurrence of *obsessions* (i.e., persistent and unwanted thoughts, images, or urges) and *compulsions* (i.e., repeated actions that are rigidly governed by internally driven rules) (Krebs & Heyman, 2015; McGowan, 2020). Although many typical children and adolescents may engage in what appear to be ritualistic behaviors and can experience obsessive thinking, it is considered a clinical diagnosis when the obsessions and compulsions cause distress, continue past an appropriate age, and begin to interfere with living life. In adolescents, these behaviors may include, but are not limited to, counting, checking, touching, washing, saying lucky words or numbers, repeating the same question, making sure things are balanced, and persisting toward an ideal or perfection (Wagner, 2009).

Since OCD can begin in adolescence, or sometimes early adulthood, engaging with a text that features teenage characters, such as *OCDaniel* by Wesley King (2016), is a great way to develop mental health literacy on this topic in the middle-level classroom. This book offers a window into the mind of Daniel, an eighth-grade boy who has symptoms of obsessive-compulsive disorder. Through Daniel's point of view, readers explore the manifestation of OCD as he experiences it throughout the story. Furthermore, in addition to the mental health component of OCD, an intriguing literacy element to follow is Daniel's journey through the age-old narrative of the hero's journey. In centering this literacy focus, students can better understand the process and essence of becoming and being a "hero."

UNDERSTANDING OBSESSIVE-COMPULSIVE DISORDER

Notably, there is a range of OCD severity, and people can present only obsessions, only compulsions, or both (Campbell, 2007). Obsessions are most often associated with fear, such as contamination or harm, while compulsions are the acts to achieve a sense of completeness, such as washing and checking (Campbell, 2007). Obsessive-compulsive disorder impacts each individual differently, so no two people present symptoms in the same way.

In terms of etiology, OCD can be passed genetically. For example, family studies looking at first-degree relatives of children and adolescents with OCD found 20–30 percent had one or more first-degree relatives with OCD, which means there are some families where siblings and/or parents have the disorder (Mattheisen et al., 2015). Understanding that OCD can have a biological basis may help students understand that mental illness is no fault of the individual. Moreover, OCD symptoms can become heightened when triggered by trauma, and the aggravation of OCD symptoms are associated with the worsening of anxiety, depressive symptoms, and avoidance behavior (Nissen et al., 2020). Obsessive-compulsive disorder can also overlap, or coexist, with other mental illnesses or medical diagnoses such as attention-deficit hyperactivity disorder, Tourette syndrome, and depression (Chaturvedi et al., 2014).

The symptoms experienced by adolescents with OCD can negatively impact their academic performance. The feeling that one needs to respond to one's obsessions and compulsions has the potential to interfere with a student's ability to pay attention, participate in discussions or presentations, study, and complete homework (Anxiety and Depression Association of America, 2020). Adolescents with OCD may also be socially withdrawn as many do not want their compulsive behaviors to be showcased or questioned (Chaturvedi et al., 2014).

Adolescents are in a stage of self-discovery—navigating peer relationships, searching for identity, learning the difference between good and evil, and dealing with the process of change, transformation, and growth—where they can relate to many aspects of the hero's journey (Cancienne, 2019). As students engage in reading *OCDaniel*, they can look to characters for models and examples to learn from, which will provide the opportunity for them to grow as readers and as citizens of the world.

OCDANIEL BY WESLEY KING

In Wesley King's (2016) *OCDaniel*, Daniel Leigh is an eighth-grader who is the back-up kicker on his high school football team; however, Daniel spends a lot of time on the bench where he counts the players, ties and reties his cleats, and rearranges the mess of cups from the team's water breaks. In fact, certain numbers are triggers for Daniel because he considers some numbers as being bad (p. 28). When Daniel is triggered, he experiences what he commonly refers to as "Zaps," or what he describes as a "pit-of-my-stomach-things-are-wrong-do-something-now feeling," but he does not fully understand why he gets them or what they are (p. 28). The Zaps are his obsessions, beginning as "the feeling of heartache" where his mind says he messed up, he'll never be happy, and he doesn't control his happiness. This makes his stomach hurt and incites the need to fix the problem or there will be harm to himself or others (pp. 49–51). These feelings come at various times, often without warning, and sometimes the Zaps lead Daniel into a place where he can't feel or think.

Daniel doesn't share his thoughts or feelings with anyone, until he meets Sara Malvern. Sara is a classmate who other students refer to as "Psycho Sara," but Daniel has always sympathized with her (p. 14). One day, Sara leaves a note in Daniel's backpack saying, "I need your help.—Fellow Star Child," which ultimately serves as the start of their friendship (p. 25). Sara shares that she's been diagnosed with "general anxiety disorder, bipolar disorder, mild schizophrenia, and depression" (p. 93). She asks for Daniel's help to find her missing father; together he and Sara find both the truth about her father and Daniel's Zaps, while Daniel plays a pivotal role on the football team as they make it to the state championship game.

GUIDING STUDENTS INTO THE TEXT

Mental Health Literacy: Obsessive-Compulsive Disorder

The title, *OCDaniel*, gives the reader the first clue that OCD will be an overarching theme of this book. Different aspects of OCD are explored throughout particular pages and chapters of the novel. For example, chapter 1 describes the process of "Zaps" for Daniel; in chapter 3, Daniel introduces the specifics on his beliefs about numbers; chapter 4 focuses on what his Routine looks like; pages 91–94 explore Sara's clinical diagnoses and Daniel asking why he is a "Star Child"; and on pages 214–16, Daniel discovers the details of obsessive-compulsive disorder.

- *Obsessive-compulsive disorder (OCD):* Obsessive-compulsive disorder is considered a chronic and long-lasting disorder that impacts a person's thoughts (obsessions) and/or behaviors (compulsions) by inciting a clinical level of repetition. Common behaviors are counting, checking, touching, and washing. Many people can display symptoms of OCD, but it becomes a concern when the obsessions and compulsions cause distress and begin to interfere with living life (Wagner, 2009).

Exploring Theme: Beginning the Hero's Journey

Before students begin reading the novel, teachers can introduce the theme of a hero's journey to provide a purpose for their reading of *OCDaniel*. There are many models for the steps and stages of the hero's journey. For this chapter, we are drawing on Campbell et al.'s

Table 8.1. Guiding Questions for Theme Identification

Act 1: Departure	Act 2: Initiation	Act 3: Return
What is the setting of the ordinary world versus the new world? What causes the character to enter the new world?	Who are the character's mentors? What trials do they encounter in the new world? Is there a major challenge they overcome?	How does the character return to the ordinary world? What has the character learned? How have they helped others?

(2014) characteristics of the hero's journey: departure, initiation, and return. *Departure* is where the character departs the ordinary after receiving a call to adventure and they enter a world with different rules where they are guided by a mentor. The character will encounter trials that test the character—thus an *initiation*—often with a major challenge they must overcome. Finally, the character *returns* to the ordinary world, where they've learned something or benefited others in a positive way.

To introduce students to the structure of the hero's journey in a story, teachers could begin by using a Pixar Short film such as *Piper* (Barrilaro, 2016) as a model. As the teacher and students view the six-minute film, they can work together to identify Campbell's three major characteristics of the hero's journey. Table 8.1 offers a list of guiding questions the teacher could pose as students identify the three characteristics of the hero's journey, and table 8.2 shows an example using *Piper* (2016).

By introducing the hero's journey prior to reading *OCDaniel* and working through an example, readers will have a model to assist them in recognizing Daniel's journey throughout the text. Reminding students

Table 8.2. Completed Graphic Organizer for the Disney Pixar Short film *Piper* (2016)

Act 1: Departure	Act 2: Initiation	Act 3: Return
Instigated by his mother, Piper, the baby sandpiper bird is pushed from the safety of his home in the sand to start finding his own food.	After getting toppled by a wave, Piper meets a sand crab who serves as his mentor. By watching the crab, he learns how to bury himself in the sand to avoid waves and he successfully forages for food.	Piper returns to the flock of sandpipers armed with his new knowledge. He can now be an adult member of the group and contribute, thus helping the flock.

that the questions are a guide for each aspect of the hero's journey will help them see beyond specifics and broadly interpret a story according to the hero's journey framework.

OCD Anticipation Guide

Before students start reading *OCDaniel*, it's important to help them distinguish between OCD misconceptions and facts. The first step a teacher could take is uncovering what students know, or believe, regarding obsessive-compulsive disorder. One way to accomplish this is through an *anticipation guide*, which will not only activate and document student understandings but also will serve as an organizer they can return to after reading the text (see figure 8.1). Once students have shared their understandings, the teacher can work through each state-

True or False?

1. Obsessive-compulsive disorder is a desire to have all belongings orderly and organized. *False*
2. People with OCD may experience uncontrollable or intrusive thoughts. *True*
3. People with OCD have obsessions with famous people or specific sports teams. *False*
4. People with OCD may have compulsions to relieve their anxious feelings. *True*
5. People with OCD often experience compulsive lying, gambling, or shopping habits. *False*
6. Doctors believe OCD is related to the biological functioning of the brain. *True*
7. People with OCD can experience it temporarily or it can last a lifetime. *True*
8. Therapy and medication can provide a reduction in OCD symptoms. *True*

Note: Correct answers are in italics following each question.
Source: Beyond OCD (2021).

Figure 8.1. Anticipation Guide for Activating Prior Knowledge of OCD

ment, providing students with the factual information needed to understand OCD as it is presented and represented in the novel.

After reading the text, students can return to this activity and complete the anticipation guide again. Students can compare their answers from before and after reading, and they can also discuss any potential misconceptions about OCD that were featured in the novel.

GUIDING STUDENTS THROUGH THE TEXT

Following Daniel on the Hero's Journey

Exploring the narrative arc of the story is a common way to lead students through and out of a novel. In addition to the typical narrative arc of setting, characters, plot, and conflict, while reading *OCDaniel* students can analyze the book through Daniel's steps of the hero's journey: departure, initiation, and return. After an incident during football, Daniel reflects that "maybe being a hero was about more than winning the game," which could be a good place to pause and discuss his journey thus far (p. 120). Students can use the provided graphic organizer (figure 8.2) to explore the theme of the hero's journey as it applies to this text. By identifying Daniel as a hero, he is viewed beyond the label of OCD, and students can see his process of growth, change, and ultimate transformation as he comes to accept his diagnosis. While Sara serves as a "mentor" to Daniel, she also experiences a transformation of her own in the structure of the hero's journey, from only being seen as "Psycho Sara" to seeking Daniel's help for her dad's mystery and ultimately becoming Daniel's support and friend.

Students can travel alongside Daniel by tracking his journey while reading the text, pausing to find textual evidence to support each aspect as listed in the graphic organizer. Although the model in figure 8.2 provides examples, there's room for student interpretation as the book is rich with subplots and story lines that follow the hero's journey framework—from Daniel's OCD, to the football team's championship run, to the mystery of Sara's father's disappearance.

Departure: Ordinary world	Departure: What causes the character to need to enter the new world?	Departure: Transitioning from the ordinary world to the new world
Daniel Leigh is an eighth grade student who is on the football team and lives at home with his mother, father, brother, and sister (chapters 1–2).	As Daniel surprisingly experiences the feelings of his "Zaps" at school, he encounters classmate Sara Malvern, who recognizes his obsessions as anxiety (p. 31). He also receives a note and follow-up email from her asking for his (p. 25 and p. 58).	Daniel's obsessions and compulsions become more severe at home, and he has a "Zaps" episode at the school dance which causes him extreme embarrassment (pp. 74–77). Sara Malvern approaches him afterwards, recognizing his embarrassment, and asking for his help to find her missing father (pp. 83–84). He becomes needed on the football team when the other kicker is injured (p. 98).
Initiation: Who are the character's mentors?	Initiation: What trials do they overcome in the new world?	Initiation: What is the major challenge they overcome?
Classmate Sara Malvern, who describes herself as a "Star Child" who is diagnosed with multiple mental illnesses (p. 93).	Daniel has various episodes of obsessions and compulsions (pp. 107–8, 115–16, 147–48, 175–77, 211–13, 227–28). Daniel learns how to be the kicker on the football team (chapters 10, 11, 13, 14, 19, 22). Daniel and Sara investigate the disappearance of Sara's father (chapters 11, 15, 17, 18, 22, 24, 25)	Daniel recognizes his counting and rituals as attempts to control his anxiety and realizes he has OCD (p. 215). Daniel's football team wins the state championship (p. 250). They discover the truth of what happened to Sara's father (p. 273).
Return: How does the character return to the ordinary world?	Return: How has the character helped others?	Return: What has the character learned?
Daniel and Sara visit the cemetery where her father is buried after learning the truth that he had passed away (p. 275). Daniel asks Sara if he can accompany her to a group therapy session (p. 287).	Daniel helps find Sara when she runs away after fighting with her mom (p. 256). He has also helped himself by connecting with someone (Sara) and sharing about his fears and anxiety (pp. 133, 192, 212, 217, 225)	Not only has Daniel learned that he has symptoms of OCD, he has accepted the idea that he might need help, that therapy could be beneficial (p. 287). While he doesn't tell his family about his obsessions or compulsions, he does feel that they would be willing to hear and accept him when he's ready (p. 290).

Figure 8.2. Completed Hero's Journey Storyboard for Daniel's Journey

The Hero's Journey Playlist

All heroes need a soundtrack. What makes music such a thoughtful representation for this novel is that two or more people can interpret and feel different things while listening to a single song, just as two or more people with symptoms or a diagnosis of a mental illness will each experience a unique journey. For this activity, students will choose songs that accompany Daniel at specific moments along his journey toward self-discovery and understanding. Students can write a two- or three-sentence explanation of how the selected song or specific song lyrics relate to an aspect of the hero's journey. Table 8.3 provides an example playlist crafted for Daniel's hero's journey toward his personal OCD discovery.

This activity provides a lot of choice and flexibility for students; they can choose various genres and songs to represent Daniel's journey while practicing the analytical skill of explaining how the song connects to the text. Students can take this further by creating a slideshow or podcast for their playlist, offering more options for using technology and sharing their product with others.

Discussion Questions

The following questions can serve as whole-class or small-group discussion questions to further an understanding of the text, or act as individual journal prompts, as students progress through the novel.

- Describe Sara Malvern. What does she understand about Daniel? Why do you think Daniel agrees to help her? What role does Sara play in terms of Daniel's hero's journey as it is portrayed in the novel? (chapter 9)
- Sara and Daniel share a connection. In what ways do they relate to each other? Why is this significant to the hero's journey? (chapter 12)
- Sara has an episode of anger and sadness regarding her father's disappearance. How does Daniel respond? Why might this be significant to his character or journey within the novel? (chapter 13)
- When Daniel's dad observes part of the Routine, how does Daniel respond? Why does he hide his feelings? Which aspect of the hero's journey can you see in this scene? (chapter 16)

Table 8.3. Completed Playlist for Daniel's Journey toward Understanding His OCD

Aspect of the Hero's Journey	Song	Artist	Explanation
Departure: Ordinary world	"Unwell"	Matchbox Twenty	This song reminds me of Daniel in the beginning of the book where he is unsure what is happening to him. The lyrics: *Hold on, feelin' like I'm headed for a breakdown* *And I don't know why* *But I'm not crazy, I'm just a little unwell*
Departure: Cause behind entering a new world	"I Want to Break Free"	Queen	Sara asks Daniel to help with her dad, so she can get answers since the mystery has been consuming her thoughts. The Zaps and the Routine get overwhelming for Daniel at times, and he finds it hard to escape them. The lyrics: *I want to break free* *I want to break free*
Departure: Transitioning from ordinary world to new world	"Better Days"	OneRepublic	The transition from feeling helpless to hopeful is this song's theme. The lyrics: *Every day is like another storm, yeah* *I'm just tryin' not to go insane* Then to lyrics: *Oh, I know that there'll be better days* *Oh, that sunshine 'bout to come my way*
Initiation: Daniel's mentor	"Most of Us Are Strangers"	Seafret	The lyrics: *Most of us are strangers* *Who want someone to save us* *We're looking out for angels* *And something we can hold on* *We are sirens, we suffer in the silence* These lyrics describe Sara and Daniel's relationship and how they both needed each other before they even knew it.

Stage	Song	Artist	Description
Initiation: Trials they overcome	"Fight Song"	Rachel Platten	Both Daniel and Sara fight through the trials they're faced with; specifically, Daniel fights through his Zaps and the challenges with being on the football team. The lyrics: *This is my fight song* / *Take back my life song*
Initiation: The major challenge Daniel overcomes	"High Hopes"	Panic! At The Disco	Daniel and Sara know it's not always easy, but they never gave up on each other, or themselves, even if it got difficult or embarrassing. The lyrics: *Stay up on that rise and never come down* / *Mama said don't give up, it's a little complicated*
Return: Returning to the ordinary world	"Control"	Zoe Wees	Daniel can connect to the following lyrics because, with Sara's help, he has a new understanding of himself and the start of having some control. The lyrics: *Tryin' every day when I hold my breath* / *Spinnin' out in space pressing on my chest* / *I don't wanna lose control* / *I need you to know, I would never be this strong without you*
Return: How Daniel helped others	"You've Got a Friend in Me"	Randy Newman	Sara played an important part in Daniel's life, but Daniel also helped Sara. He helped with the mystery of her dad but also acted as a friend when he was in need. The lyrics: *You've got a friend in me* / *You've got troubles, I've got 'em too* / *There isn't anything I wouldn't do for you*
Return: What Daniel has learned	"On Top of the World"	Imagine Dragons	The book ends with Daniel being able to delay the Routine, and he realizes he is normal; he comes to understand that "normal" isn't just one way of being, it is when a person can be themselves and express themselves, which makes Daniel feel good about himself. He also doesn't feel alone anymore. The lyrics: *I'm on top of the world, 'ey* / *Waiting on this for a while now*

- When Sara admits to seeing Daniel's nighttime routine through the window, he confesses to his difficulties. Why do you think he tells Sara? Think about her role in his journey. (chapter 19)
- Daniel says to Sara, "Maybe I'm being punished for not being a good kid all the time or something" (p. 212). How do you think Daniel altering this thinking can influence his development through his hero's journey? (chapter 19)
- Daniel connects to the characteristics of OCD outlined in the book Sara gives him. How does this affect his self-image? How does this play a role in his journey? (chapter 20)
- Sara confronts Daniel about his discovery of his obsessive-compulsive disorder. Why won't he tell anyone about it? (chapter 20)
- What is the truth of Sara's father's disappearance? How does Sara experience aspects of her own hero's journey in her discovery of the truth? (chapter 25)
- Daniel expresses interest in joining Sara for her therapy group. How has Daniel changed since discovering his Zaps are part of a disorder called obsessive-compulsive disorder? Connect his growth to his hero's journey. (chapter 27)

GUIDING STUDENTS OUT OF THE TEXT

A Call to Action

Studies have found that those with mental illness who experience discrimination, rejection, and/or stigmatization can have a poorer quality of life (Sickel et al., 2014). People who advocate for de-stigmatization or model appropriate, accepting behavior can create positive change for those with mental health issues or illness. With each other's support, both Daniel and Sara begin to change the way they feel about themselves after both having used traditionally negative words at separate times to describe themselves. Daniel thinks he might be crazy when he talks about his numbers, Sara calls herself "certifiably nuts," and Daniel believes he is imbalanced (pp. 29, 93, 116).

Open Your Mind to Mental Illness

The main objective of this activity is for students to consider the perspective of a character or person with mental illness. For this activity, teachers can give students a blank copy of an "open mind" (figure 8.3), or they can draw one themselves. The mind will be split in half: one half will represent what Sara or Daniel might be feeling or thinking at the conclusion of the novel, and the other half will be what the other characters featured in this novel or society can do to open their minds to Sara or Daniel's experiences. Students can use words, symbols, drawings, or pictures to represent the thoughts and feelings of the character. A written piece accompanies the open mind where the students write to explain why they chose each picture or symbol.

An open mind activity is a perspective-taking activity and helps students employ empathy when thinking about the challenges a character is facing. This activity can be equally powerful when looking at Daniel

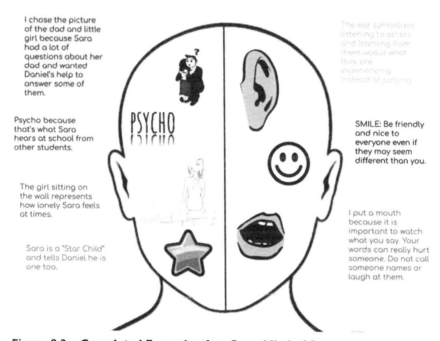

I chose the picture of the dad and little girl because Sara had a lot of questions about her dad and wanted Daniel's help to answer some of them.

Psycho because that's what Sara hears at school from other students.

The girl sitting on the wall represents how lonely Sara feels at times.

Sara is a "Star Child" and tells Daniel he is one too.

The ear symbolizes listening to others and learning from them about what they are experiencing instead of judging

SMILE: Be friendly and nice to everyone even if they may seem different than you.

I put a mouth because it is important to watch what you say. Your words can really hurt someone. Do not call someone names or laugh at them.

Figure 8.3. Completed Example of an Open Mind of Sara

or Sara; perhaps partnering students together while one completes one character's open mind and the other completes the other character's open mind could allow for a compare and contrast view of their experiences.

Combating Stigma with a "Just Because" Poem

In the text, Daniel faces the fear of what people will think of him, as evidenced by his reluctance to talk to anyone about his obsessions and compulsions. He doesn't want to be stereotyped for being different, and he hides his friendship with Sara because she is negatively stereotyped by other people at school. Students can create a "Just Because" poem for a character in *OCDaniel*. The general format of a "Just Because" poem, as highlighted in figure 8.4, explores the misconceptions of the stereotype through non-rhyming verse, with questions and a statement of positive understanding at the end.

"Just Because" poems are helpful for overcoming stereotypes or personal insecurities. It allows students to practice changing mind-sets and attitudes about things that are traditionally viewed as negative.

Just because I'm diagnosed with OCD
It doesn't mean I'm out of control,
Doesn't mean I'm organizing all of my belongings,
And it doesn't mean I can't join in regular activities.
Just because I'm diagnosed with OCD,
It doesn't mean I'm unable to function,
Doesn't mean I can't be in regular classes in school,
And doesn't mean I can't play football.
And just because I have OCD
Why should people treat me like I'm not normal?
Who says I can't lead a healthy, typical life?
When will others realize the seriousness of mental health?
I have OCD and I will be okay.

Figure 8.4.   Example "Just Because" Poem for Daniel

Closing the Book

Reading the author's note aloud with students allows that personal connection between the character and the writer. *OCDaniel* is an #ownvoices text (Corinne Duyvis, n.d.), where the author shares the OCD diagnosis of the protagonist. The author gives personal insight into his own adolescent experiences, including navigating mental illness in isolation until he was 16 years old. To process the author's note, teachers can consider posting the author's note in short chunks on chart paper around the classroom in a setup similar to a museum viewing. Teachers can then encourage students to have a "silent dialogue" with the text. A small group of students can gather around each chart paper and use markers to respond to each section of the text. Students can respond by writing questions, comments, or connections; the goal is to have an interaction with the text through their writing. After a few minutes, students can rotate to the next chart paper and continue the silent dialogue by reading the next chunk of text and responding with their marker on the paper. As the activity progresses, students can respond to each other's comments on the chart paper. The order of the text isn't overly important; the students will read the author's note in its entirety by the time they complete the activity. The strategy of a "silent dialogue" provides space for every student to share their voice through writing. It can be a way for students to process challenging information before discussing it aloud. The teacher could invite a school counselor to join the conversation and facilitate a verbal discussion on the comments and questions shared within the students' written dialogue.

CONCLUSION

Eighth grader Daniel Leigh narrates his journey of experiencing obsessions and compulsions, and keeping them secret from his family, friends, and teachers. By the end of the text, Daniel's journey comes to a close on various fronts: his football team wins the state championship with his help, he assists Sara in discovering what happened to her father, and he comes to accept his Zaps and Routine as features of obsessive-compulsive disorder. Though Daniel's experience follows the *departure*, *initiation*, and *return* aspects of the hero's journey, his journey is not yet complete. Although he hasn't yet formally sought help or support from his family or a trusted professional, readers leave him wanting to attend a therapy session, being able to delay the Routine, and feeling better about possibly sharing his experiences with his family. As the author, Wesley King (2016), says in his dedication of the book to those diagnosed with OCD, "hope is rarely found alone" (p. v). While Daniel does find Sara who provides him some support in discovering his disorder, it is crucial that students walk away with the message that help is available and it is okay to talk to a trusted adult; as Daniel finally realizes at the end, he wouldn't be alone anymore.

REFERENCES

American Psychiatric Association. (2013). *Diagnostic and statistical manual of mental disorders* (5th ed.). Washington, DC: American Psychiatric Publishing. https://doi.org/10.1176/appi.books.9780890425596

Anxiety and Depression Association of America. (2020). *OCD at school*. https://adaa.org/understanding-anxiety/obsessive-compulsive-disorder/ocd-at-school

Barrilaro, A. (Director). (2016). *Piper* [Film]. Pixar Animation Studios.

Beyond OCD. (2021). *What is OCD and how is it recognized?* BeyondOCD .org. https://beyondocd.org/ocd-facts/what-is-ocd

Campbell, J., Cousineau, P., & Brown, S. L. (2014). *The hero's journey: Joseph Campbell on his life and work (The collected works of Joseph Campbell)* (3rd ed.). Novato, CA: New World Library.

Campbell, N. (2007, February 9). Clinical: How you can identify OCD symptoms. *GP*, 42. https://link.gale.com/apps/doc/A159018918/GPS?u=fairfaxcps &sid=GPS&xid=3e4f3814

Cancienne, M. B. (2019). Using metaphorical thinking to understand a literary archetype: The hero's journey. *Virginia English Journal*, 69(1), 59–71.

Chaturvedi, A., Murdick, N. L., & Gartin, B. C. (2014). Obsessive compulsive disorder: What an educator needs to know. *Physical Disabilities: Education and Related Services*, 33(2), 71–83. https://doi.org/10.14434/pders.v33i2.13134

Corinne Duyvis [@corinneduyvis]. (n.d.). *Tweets* [Twitter profile]. Twitter. Retrieved April 23, 2021, from https://twitter.com/corinneduyvis?ref_src =twsrc%5Egoogle%7Ctwcamp%5Eserp%7Ctwgr%5Eauthor

King, W. (2016). *OCDaniel*. New York: Simon & Schuster.

Krebs, G., & Heyman, I. (2015). Obsessive-compulsive disorder in children and adolescents. *Archives of Disease in Childhood, 100*(5), 495–99. https:// doi.org/10.1136/archdischild-2014-306934

Mattheisen, M., Samuels, J. F., Wang, Y., Greenberg, B. D., Fyer, A. J., Mc-Cracken, J. T., & Nestadt, G. (2015). Genome-wide association study in obsessive-compulsive disorder: Results from the OCGAS. *Molecular Psychiatry, 20*(3), 337–44. https://doi.org/10.1038/mp.2014.43

McGowan, H. (2020). Pediatric OCD: A case for vigilance. *Pediatric News, 54*(6), 10. https://link.gale.com/apps/doc/A629397709/GPS?u=fairfaxcps&sid =GPS&xid=c28d1035

Nissen, J. B., Hajgaard, D. R. M. A., & Thomsen, P. H. (2020). The immediate effect of COVID-19 pandemic on children and adolescents with obsessive compulsive disorder. *BMC Psychiatry, 20*, 511. https://doi.org/10.1186/ s12888-020-02905-5

Sickel, A. E., Seacat, J. D., & Nabors, N. A. (2014). Mental health stigma update: A review of consequences. *Advances in Mental Health, 12*(3), 202–15. https://doi.org/10.1080/18374905.2014.11081898

Wagner, A. P. (2009). *Obsessive-compulsive disorder in children and adolescents*. International OCD Foundation. https://iocdf.org/wp-content/up loads/2014/10/OCD-in-Children-and-Teenagers-Fact-Sheet.pdf

EXPLORING MENTAL HEALTH LITERACY THROUGH BOOK CLUBS

Lesley Roessing and Jessica Traylor

Book clubs are an effective way to facilitate discussions about topics related to mental health issues. Given that one in six children have a diagnosed mental health condition (Centers for Disease Control, 2020), the experiences of fictional characters can touch on concerns that many students have personally experienced or have witnessed in their family or friends. Knowing how to hold conversations about sensitive issues serves students well, not only in class but also in other areas of life.

Reading about and discussing a variety of mental health issues supports students in developing mental health literacy. When students are able to recognize the symptoms of mental distress, learn how to seek help, and hold attitudes that reduce stigma, they are more likely to seek treatment early and can be better equipped to support their friends (Furnham & Swami, 2018; Wilder, 2019). Regarding mental health, early recognition and intervention are key to reducing the potential negative consequences. The ability to discuss symptoms of a variety of mental health issues in the lives of multiple fictional characters, develop empathy for these characters, and see them seek and receive help can support students in moving toward constructive ideas about mental health issues (Furnham & Swami, 2018; Sevinc, 2019).

CHOOSING THE BOOK CLUB SELECTIONS

Any of the novels in this collection would be effective for combining into book clubs; however, there are five novels offered as examples for the book club reading described in this chapter: *Scars* (Rainfield, 2010), *Saving Red* (Sones, 2016), *Wintergirls* (Anderson, 2009), *The Unlikely Hero of Room 13B* (Toten, 2013), and *The Memory of Light* (Stork, 2017).

These novels were selected with a mind-set of including a variety of mental health issues, a variety of writing formats, lengths, and narrative complexity, a diversity of reading levels, cultural diversity of characters and authors (diversity is defined as ethnicity, race, age, geography/nationality, gender identification, sexual orientation), and novels that are #ownvoices writings by authors who have experience with mental health issues, either personally or through family members (Corinne Duyvis, n.d.).

SETTING UP THE BOOK CLUBS

The first step for implementing book club reading is to divide the members of the class into book clubs, each reading a different novel. The novels should guide the composition of the book clubs, rather than vice versa. Readers will be working with these books for three to four weeks; therefore, group members should be reading texts they *can* read and *will* read, supported by other readers who are also interested in that text. Before choosing a book, the teacher can give a short book talk about each of the selections, telling the students a little about the themes, plot, setting, characters, and the author.

Students each select a novel, examine the front and back covers, and read one or two pages. The teacher can discuss the importance of reading a few pages, explaining that readers may be interested in the topic or title, be intrigued by any cover art, and be engaged by the synopsis but may not find the author's writing style appealing or may find the writing or vocabulary too challenging or not challenging enough. After two or three minutes, each student selects and considers another novel until they have examined all five novels and made their choices.

The students write down their first, second, and third choices. It is effective to have them write down a reason why they want to read a particular text, as it causes the readers to reflect on their choices and allows teachers to recognize reasons that may not be apparent for matching a student with a book. For example, a reader with background knowledge about a mental health issue, either from personal experience or prior research, may be able to read a novel of a higher reading level as their background knowledge of a topic can enhance their comprehension of the text. Also, reader interest in a topic or a character can increase reading motivation (Roessing, 2007, 2019). Teachers can guide student reflections by asking students to think about *why* they may have an interest in a particular book choice and give some examples of how they choose books to read.

The teacher can then look over the students' choices and divide the students into clubs, providing as many students as possible the opportunity to read one of their top choices. This method allows the teacher to privately determine if students have chosen texts that may be too challenging or not challenging enough as first choices and, if so, to assign the second or third more appropriate choice (Roessing, 2019).

ORGANIZING BOOK CLUB READING AND MEETINGS

Ideally, the book club structure allows time for both reading and meeting discussions, guided by short focus lessons presented by the teacher. A typical Reading Workshop format has five elements:

- A read-aloud of a short mentor text
- A 10- or 15-minute focus lesson on a reading literacy element or, in this case, a mental health literacy element
- A block of time for independent reading and reading reflection journaling or notes for the next meeting
- Teacher conferences with individual students during the independent reading time
- A final sharing of how the literacy lesson was applied during the reading

Classes reading in book clubs can follow the same basic format with modifications. For example, in 45- or 60-minute classes, teachers can alternate between Reading Days and Book Club Meeting Days. The typical Reading Workshop format described in the last paragraph can be followed on Reading Days. On Meeting Days, the workshop format would follow an adapted plan:

- Reference to the Mentor Text Read-Aloud from the correlated Reading Day
- A 10-minute focus lesson that provides a discussion topic for the meeting
- A 25-minute book club meeting
- A 10-minute interclub meeting

If the class follows a 90-minute block schedule, both meeting and reading opportunities could take place within the same period every other day.

Prior to reading and discussing their novels, the teacher can facilitate one or two class periods of Mental Health Literacy Pre-reading Lessons to prepare students for the types of symptoms, stressors, and supports they will encounter in their novels and a class period of Reading Literacy Pre-reading Lessons to prepare students for reflective journaling and book club discussion techniques.

READING LITERACY PRE-READING LESSONS

If students have not been trained in reader response journaling, the teacher can teach the purpose of reader response, which is reader reflection, compelling readers to explore, question, and challenge text and make connections and inferences so they can construct meaning and learn from text to increase comprehension (Roessing, 2009). Written reader response also provides notes for book club discussions and for assessment purposes so teachers can see if, what, and how readers are reading independently.

Teachers can introduce simple response starters, such as "A question I have," "I wonder why," "What I found most interesting," and practice

5-minute responses with a narrative poem. Teachers can introduce a double-entry response journal and model journaling with such a form during the Reading Literacy Focus Lessons based on a mentor text as described in the following section.

Teachers can also lead a short lesson on discussion skills, such as the criteria for designing effective discussion questions to engage conversation, setting community conversation norms and methods for expanding a conversation or respectful disagreement prior to beginning book club reading.

MENTAL HEALTH LITERACY PRE-READING LESSONS

Mental health is a broad topic that can cover a variety of thoughts, feelings, and behaviors. Knowing the symptoms of mental illness, seeking treatment when needed, and being open to mental health support are important in addressing mental illness and maintaining mental health. Successful coping can result in improved resilience, even in the face of seemingly overwhelming situations.

The first Mental Health Literacy Pre-reading Lesson provides students with basic background information on mental health. It is important for students to understand that mental health is like physical health; there are times in a person's life when they feel healthier than others; experiencing mental health difficulties can be a normal response to difficult situations.

This first Mental Health Pre-reading Lesson offers a framework for viewing mental health literacy, consisting of four general areas: knowledge of mental health issues, erroneous beliefs and stereotypes, help-seeking behavior, and self-help strategies. Another option for addressing knowledge of mental health issues is to present data about the prevalence of mental illness in the nation, state, or local community.

The second Mental Health Pre-reading Lesson narrows the focus to a discussion of previous experiences with or ideas about mental health and mental health concerns. This naturally leads to a discussion of stereotypes about mental illness and knowledge of mental health supports and self-help strategies. The following questions can be used to guide the discussion:

1. How do mental health conditions affect a person's thoughts, feelings, and behaviors?
2. How do general health behaviors—like adequate sleep, healthy eating, consistent exercise, and stress reduction—contribute to mental health?
3. How can friends and family be helpful to a person with a mental health condition?
4. What are the advantages of seeking professional help from a counselor, social worker, psychologist, or psychiatrist?
5. What are some common stigmas, stereotypes, or misconceptions about mental health conditions or about people with mental health conditions?

The goal of facilitating a discussion about mental health issues is to encourage students to begin thinking about these factors. By discussing their existing knowledge, students can begin to think about the stressors, symptoms, and supports they may encounter in the novels.

READING LITERACY FOCUS LESSONS

On each reading or book club meeting day, class begins with a mentor text, in this case a short story that will be used as the mentor text for all the Reading Literacy and Mental Health Literacy lessons.

Teachers can encourage readers to reflect on the day's focus lesson in their reading response notes taken during or after reading and bring their notes to the following book club meeting. Students can use a double-sided, double-entry journal such as the one featured in figure 9.1 for their reader response notes.

Francisco Stork's 2018 short story "Captain, My Captain" is an example of a mentor text that teachers can effectively employ for both literacy and mental health focus lessons. This is the first-person narrative of Alberto, a Latino boy who lives with his sister and her baby and has dropped out of high school to work and send money to his family in Mexico. He was diagnosed with "intellectual and developmental disabilities" (Stork, 2018, p.174). Alberto hears a voice in his head, which he refers to as Captain America, that prescribes his actions, especially to leave his sister's abusive relationship. Alberto's friend Becky encourages him to seek support from a therapist who has helped her.

The Reading Workshop begins with a short focus lesson, pointing readers to elements that increase comprehension, lead proficient readers to even deeper understanding of the text, and facilitate discussion about these novels. While teachers can choose any concept to teach through a focus lesson, in this case, concepts should be those (1) influenced by or influencing the mental health issues introduced in the novels and (2) that apply to all the book club novels.

For the first Reading Literacy Lesson, however, it would be advantageous for teachers to focus on point of view with the objective of having readers note from whose perspective the narrative is told and, for more critical reading, determining how the point of view affects the story and impacts the reader's opinion of characters and events. Teachers should guide readers to contextualize the perspective of the narrator in first-person narration.

Reading the first five pages of the mentor text "Captain, My Captain" (pp. 157–62), teachers can think aloud and identify the point of view as third-person limited. Teachers can reflect that a narrator is telling the story in third person by referring to Alberto as "he," but the perspective is limited to one character, Alberto. The reader learns what Alberto thinks, feels, and perceives; the perspective is almost as restricted as first person, but the narration is not in Alberto's voice.

The teacher might question that, if Alberto hears a voice, might that reflect the possibility that this may be the reason the author wrote in third-person limited—so that readers could have insight into what Alberto was thinking and follow a counternarrative? While reading these initial pages, teachers can stop and reflect aloud on what they, as readers, know and what they learn about Alberto as a consequence of the perspective. Teachers may reflect on other advantages and disadvantages of third-person narration. Teachers could consider how this literary point of view lets the reader assume that Captain America is not a real person.

As they begin to read the first section of their novels, teachers can ask readers to note the point of view through which their story is told and the various ways this point of view affects, or may affect, the story and their reading of it, as the teacher did in the model lesson.

For these particular novels, it would be appropriate to maintain a continuing lesson on character relationships. Peer relationships can be simple and supportive and even life-saving or can be complex, antagonistic, or even toxic. Peer relationships are central in adolescent life and even more significant for an adolescent suffering from mental illness (Holman et al., 2019); family relationships can also affect adolescents and can impact mental health (Furnham & Swami, 2018).

In the literacy focus lessons, as teachers read through the mentor text, they can reflect on Alberto's past relationships with his parents and his current, evolving relationships with Captain America, Lupe, Wayne, and Becky, and the ways each relationship appears to affect his goals and his mental health.

As students begin to read assigned sections of their novels and prepare for their book club meetings, they can note the main characters' relationships in the section they are reading. In each reading, they will analyze how these relationships are developing and identify connections with any new characters. The second page of the Book Club Double-Entry Journal (see figure 9.1) includes sections for these reflections.

It is also important for readers to consider minor characters' relationships to each other and how those relationships may affect the protagonists and their goals and decisions. Reading Literacy Lessons are paired with Mental Health Literacy Lessons to lead readers to deeper reading, more profound comprehension, and enhanced book club meeting discussions.

MENTAL HEALTH LITERACY FOCUS LESSONS

Mental Health Literacy Lessons can be interspersed with the Reading Literacy Lessons delineated earlier and will highlight the interactions between the characters, specifically related to symptoms of mental illness and other sub-clinical mental health concerns. Teachers can encourage readers to look for thoughts, feelings, and/or behaviors that influence the relationships between characters. Sometimes these thoughts, feelings, and behaviors will elicit positive, supportive interaction, but sometimes the reader may notice resulting interactions that are

Name _____ Novel _____

Mental Heath Lteracy BOOK CLUB Double-Entry Journal

For Meeting Date _____ Chapters _____ to _____ Pages _____ to _____

Summary—list the main events from the chapters read in bullet points, highlight new characters

- _____
- _____
- _____
- _____
- _____
- _____
- _____
- _____
- _____
- _____

Discussion Question #1 about the narrative:

_____

_____

_____

_____

Discussion Question #2 based on the Mental Health Literacy Lesson:

_____

_____

_____

_____

Figure 9.1.   Mental Health Literacy Book Club Double-Entry Journal

(*continued*)

From the TEXT:	My THOUGHTS about what I read:
1. Based on the topic of current Focus Lesson	My Thoughts and Reflections
2. Something the Character Says or Does	My Thoughts and Reflections
3. Relationship(s) between Character(s)	My Thoughts and Reflections
4. An Event from the Text	My Inference or Prediction based on that Event

Figure 9.1. *Continued*

unsupportive or harmful. Teachers can include lessons that focus on the ways in which supporting characters encourage the main character to seek professional help or provide some other form of support.

Teachers should have a mental health professional available to help facilitate these discussions. School counselors, social workers, and psychologists could serve this important role. These mental health professionals not only offer specialized knowledge, but also their presence in the classroom could serve to acknowledge and support the idea that talking with mental health professionals can be a natural part of maintaining mental health.

While reading the mentor text, teachers can model the process of thinking about how signs of mental or emotional distress play a role in Alberto's relationships. Thinking aloud, teachers talk about the impact of stress on relationship dynamics, especially the distress caused by competing expectations from others, for instance, the expectations of Lupe and Wayne. Teachers could also mention the effect of Captain America on Alberto's ability to fulfill his obligations to his family. Students can look for similar relationship dynamics in their own novels.

After reading "Captain, My Captain," teachers can reflect on how the other characters supported Alberto. In addition to the environment created by Alberto's relationships, the teacher can reflect on how living with Lupe and Wayne could have affected Alberto's mental and emotional health.

Alberto received informal support from Lupe and Becky. Noticing that Becky's relationship with Alberto was instrumental in his decision to seek professional help, teachers can discuss how friends can be sources of support during one's treatment seeking and engagement, remission, or ongoing difficulties.

Students will be prepared to observe a variety of effects that relationships can have in preparing for their book club discussions. Being able to recognize and discuss these elements in their novels can support more critical reading and the development of greater mental health literacy.

THE NOVELS

Scars by Cheryl Rainfield (2010)

Summary

It has been three years since the abuse ended; it has been six months since 15-year-old Kendra started remembering the abuse she suffered since she was a toddler. As flashbacks of the sexual abuse surface, Kendra can remember everything except the identity of her abuser. She is certain he is following her, especially when she finds threatening notes left for her. Cutting helps her relieve her building anxiety.

Kendra also finds relief through her art even though her artist mother disapproves of her methods. Luckily, Kendra is receiving support from Carolyn, her empathetic therapist, her art teacher who is studying art therapy, and Meghan, a new girlfriend who is struggling through her own family issues.

Mental health issues: Posttraumatic stress disorder (PTSD), self-harm, sexual abuse.

Why the Novel Was Chosen

The author, a queer female, is an abuse survivor, and the mental health issues and their complexity are authentically portrayed in the novel. The main character, an abuse survivor, and two supporting characters are also queer. The novel tackles sexual abuse, abuse survival, cutting, anxiety, trauma, therapies, family relationships, homophobia, and lesbian relationships. This novel portrays a positive exploration of mental health services and ends with a plan for recovery, rather than a quick fix.

Look-Fors Based on Reading Literacy Lessons

Although the story is told from Kendra's point of view, the relationships among the characters are interesting to note. For example, the interactions between the mother and each of the other characters are very complicated although Kendra does not appear a complex character herself. Notably, although Kendra's mother is homophobic, her friend

Sandy is a gay man, and she admits to conflicted responses and a willing-ness to expand her perspective.

The relationship between Kendra and Carolyn is compassionate, and it will be interesting for readers to note when Carolyn crosses, ap-propriately, the therapist-patient relationship and how this additionally supports Kendra and her recovery. Also, as a queer character who has come out and survived a previous but injurious relationship, students can consider how this experience might influence Kendra's new rela-tionship with Meghan.

Look-Fors Based on Mental Health Literacy Lessons

Kendra's symptoms are primarily revealed through flashbacks and internal thoughts. Students can discuss how Kendra's flashbacks are intrusive, cause distress, and result in difficulties functioning at school and home. Becoming aware of symptoms of mental health difficulties is an important aspect of developing mental health literacy (Furnham & Swami, 2018). Beyond flashbacks and cutting, Kendra also exhibits physical symptoms.

Attitudes about mental health issues are a primary factor in the choice to seek help. Students can discuss Kendra's attitude toward fully en-gaging in counseling, especially regarding whether she should disclose her symptoms to the counselor. Students can also discuss Kendra's relationship with her parents and other secondary characters. The ways that Kendra's symptoms interfere with her relationships and ability to be honest with others could offer significant discussion opportunities. Readers can discuss various types of support provided by Carolyn, Ms. Archer, and Meghan throughout the novel.

Saving Red by Sonya Sones (2016)

Summary

While completing a high school service project, 14-year-old Molly meets Red, a homeless 18-year-old girl, and they become friends. Molly makes it her mission to reunite Red with her family and, after realizing that Red suffers from mental illness, to keep her safe. Molly has her own issues with anxiety and guilt, alleviated by Pixel, her service dog.

In addition, Molly's brother suffered from PTSD and has been missing since leaving home a year ago.

Mental health issues: Schizoaffective disorder, PTSD, anxiety—specifically panic disorder. Although Molly's diagnosis is not officially named in the text, the author alludes to the symptoms of anxiety and references panic attacks.

Why the Novel Was Chosen

The novel is written in free verse, which is a variation from the other four novels selected for these book clubs. The main character, Molly, is Jewish, and some Jewish cultural traditions are included in the novel.

The novel also demonstrates the efficacy of mental health services and the importance of discussion and advocacy. The author has personal experience with mental illness; her older sister was diagnosed with bipolar disorder when she was 13 years old.

Look-Fors Based on Reading Literacy Lessons

The story is told from Molly's perspective in first person. This is essential as the reader experiences Red from Molly's point of view, revealing Red's mental health issues over time. Molly discusses her anxiety, but readers are not certain of the source until she shares her story with Red; readers learn the reasons her family has become so dysfunctional only when Molly confronts her parents.

The characters and the relationships among them are also interpreted by Molly. Readers will want to analyze her need for her friendship with Red and her new friend Cristo, as well as discuss how the loss of her relationship with her brother has affected her and her decisions.

Look-Fors Based on Mental Health Literacy Lessons

The reader is exposed to Molly's stereotypes about mental illness the first time she sees Red. Students can discuss Molly's initial thoughts about how her attitude changed throughout time. Molly's initial interactions with Cristo and her expectations about his judgment of Red could also serve as a basis for discussion regarding stereotypes. Students can further consider the effect of negative attitudes about mental health issues and help seeking on Red's reluctance to accept handouts from Molly or spend the night in a homeless shelter.

Molly and Red's relationship provides the foundation for the novel. Some students may wonder if the relationship between Molly and Red would have existed without Molly's grief and guilt over the disappearance of her brother. Students may also want to discuss how Molly's relationships with Pixel and Cristo often served to calm her symptoms of anxiety.

Environmental stressors and supports are abundant in the novel. While not often in the forefront, readers can discuss Molly's relationship with her parents, especially regarding the effect of her parents' dysfunctional coping behaviors on their ability to provide support for Molly.

Students can discuss the support Molly tries to provide for Red, specifically regarding food, shelter, and clothing. Additionally, Cristo's emotional and material support play an important role in Molly's ability to "save" Red. The availability of and attitudes toward mental health services and medication by the characters could also provide useful material for discussion.

Wintergirls by Laurie Halse Anderson (2009)

Summary

Lia comes from a dysfunctional family. She is a person who is engaging in anorexic behaviors; she counts every single calorie and cannot reach a "perfect" weight. After spending time in rehab, Lia is not better; she just hides her disordered eating behaviors better. Before their friendship ended, Lia and Cassie were best friends who made a pact to be the skinniest. When Lia realizes that Cassie called her 33 times on the night she died—alone in a hotel room, she begins seeing visions of Cassie's spirit, goading her to join her in death. Finally, Lia's actions affect not only her own life but also that of her younger half sister, and she finds out how Cassie really died.

Mental health issues: Symptoms of anorexia, symptoms of bulimia, cutting, visions, hallucinations.

Why the Novel Was Chosen

The author is well known among teachers and students, possibly lead-ing readers to choose this novel to read. Anderson is able to communi-cate the addictive power of anorexia and anorexic behaviors. The author conferred with a pediatrician and a psychotherapist who are experts in the field. Most important, eating disorders are on the rise. The National Institute of Mental Health (2017) reports that 2.7 percent of teens, ages 13–18, struggle with an eating disorder. In one study of adolescent girls, 5.2 percent of the girls met criteria for anorexia, bulimia, or binge eating disorder. And young people between the ages of 15 and 24 with anorexia have 10 times the risk of dying compared to their same-aged peers (National Eating Disorders Association, 2020). The story endorses the importance of treatment for eating disorders.

Look-Fors Based on Reading Literacy Lessons

The story is told from Cassie's point of view. Readers view the other characters through Cassie's eyes, which is important as this is how she experiences the world. Readers also experience food as someone with anorexia might perceive it: calorie by calorie.

Students can analyze the many complex relationships in the story, including Lia's relationships with Cassie, her mother, her father, Jenni-fer, her younger sister, Elijah, her therapist, and Lia's own relationship with food. They can discuss healthy and unhealthy relationships and ways these relationships change and evolve over the course of the novel. Lia's goals and motivations are driven by her mental health struggles, which also provide the obstacles to her goals. Book club discussions will most likely address the ways in which Lia's goals change as she further engages in treatment.

Lia changes how she navigates problems throughout the novel as she interacts with others and gains more information about Cassie. Book club members can discuss their interpretations of why and how Lia makes decisions, such as her decision to visit the room where Cassie died, her decision to finally talk to her therapist, and her decision on whether to get help.

Look-Fors Based on Mental Health Literacy Lessons

Symptoms of anorexia are present from the first time Jennifer, Lia's stepmother, encourages her to eat breakfast. Readers can discuss Lia's distress when her thoughts shift between eating or not eating, as well as the fact that she feels strong when she is empty. Although the reader experiences Lia's body deteriorating, Lia continues to think that strict calorie restriction is a sign of strength. The impact Lia's symptoms have on Emma can lead to a productive discussion of how mental health concerns affect the whole family.

This novel can lead readers to a discussion of the common American sociocultural stereotype that "skinny is good." Lia and Cassie both suffer because of their belief in this stereotype. Lia's primary goal is to lose weight. Regardless of her weight, she continues to set the bar lower. Readers can discuss how each decision Lia makes supports this goal and leads her farther away from her support system.

Students may discuss how Lia's family dynamic contributes to her mental and emotional distress. For instance, her mother's clinical approach, her father's absence, and her sister's admiration all play a role in the development and eventual treatment of anorexia. Lia lives with her father and stepmother; however, her father is rarely present. Lia's mother lives in the home Lia grew up in, but it has been completely remodeled. Readers can discuss how Lia feels about the dynamics in these two home environments. They can note and discuss the balance of structure, nurturing, and attention Lia receives and how those factors could affect the course of her mental and emotional development.

Lia's relationship with Cassie could be noted and discussed as a significant factor because they mutually reinforced each other for their unhealthy eating behaviors. Readers may also note that Lia is relatively isolated from her peer group, which could lead to discussion of how mental health difficulties can result in withdrawing from social life.

Lia's relationship with her therapist, Dr. Parker, changes during the course of the novel with Lia eventually being honest about the severity of her symptoms. Readers could note and discuss Lia's role in her own recovery throughout the novel. Realizing the importance of Lia's choice to actively participate in treatment can offer significant insight for readers.

The Unlikely Hero of Room13B by Teresa Toten (2013)

Summary

Fourteen-year-old Adam Spencer Ross belongs to a young adult obsessive-compulsive disorder (OCD) support group. When he meets and instantly falls in love with the newest member, Robyn Plummer, recently released from a residential facility, he decides he will get better, save Robyn, and become the superhero that he has chosen as his group identity. Complicating this, Adam has two families, one composed of a detached father and a loving stepmother, and, the other, an anxiety-filled younger half brother and his mother who demonstrates hoarding tendencies with additional mental health issues. Adam tries navigating his world, suppressing his OCD, working with his therapist, and helping those around him. Adam's story highlights the importance of family, friendship, and hope in the treatment of mental health issues.

Mental health issues: Obsessive-compulsive disorder, hoarding, possible substance abuse.

Why the Novel Was Chosen

This novel includes a male protagonist and three other male characters and three female characters in his adolescent therapy group, as well as their Jamaican therapist, Chuck. *Unlikely Hero* demonstrates different manifestations of a mental health issue, in this case OCD, with characters who display various severities and symptoms of OCD and are at different stages of acknowledging and working to mitigate the effects of this disorder. The story highlights the advantages of group therapy, private therapy sessions, and residential treatment as well as the hope for recovery.

Look-Fors Based on Reading Literacy Lessons

Unlikely Hero is narrated in third-person limited, offering a different discussion from the three novels discussed earlier. Adam lies a lot, and readers can discuss how first-person narration would affect the story and what the reader knows at different points in the story.

The novel begins with a group session, and readers are introduced to the adolescents and Adam's therapist; the family situations are introduced during the course of the novel. Adam's goal, to win the love of Robyn, and the obstacle, his mental health issues, are made clear immediately, but students can identify other goals, and obstacles, as the novel progresses. Adam's decisions can generate important conversations about adolescence, mental health, and family.

The relationship between Adam and the other characters (i.e., Robyn, the group, his therapist, his mother, his father, Sweetie) becomes more complex as Adam gains knowledge about each of them.

Look-Fors Based on Mental Health Literacy Lessons

Readers are introduced to Adam's OCD diagnosis during the first group meeting. Throughout the novel, readers will notice counting, cleaning, and tapping. Like many individuals with mental illness, Adam is aware of his symptoms and tries to suppress them in public, especially in the presence of Robyn.

Several common stereotypes are encountered during this novel. The group visits a Catholic church and is initially met with awkward glances from the priest. The reader will notice Adam's response to Father Rick, "we're not violent," during his group's visit to the church, as a response to the concern they may be perceived as dangerous due to their group identification (p. 168). While Adam would like to gain more control over his obsessive thoughts and compulsive behaviors, his goal is accelerated when he meets Robyn. Readers can note and discuss the shift in Adam's active effort to participate in his treatment.

Adam's family relationships are significant sources of stress and support. His mother's hoarding and substance use cause increased stress, as evidenced by the increasing difficulty Adam has entering his front door. His relationship with Sweetie, while stressful, also gives Adam a reason to seek help and gain a level of insight into how his rituals could have developed. Sharing his strategies with Sweetie and reflecting on their usefulness throughout the novel is an outward manifestation of Adam's changing thoughts about his disorder.

Adam's family relationships take place across different environments. His mother's home is cluttered and leads to increased anxiety, while his father's home is clean, nurturing, and supportive of his treatment. Beyond Adam's family relationships, readers will notice the relationship dynamics between Adam and his therapist and each of his group members. Outside of the family dynamics, Robyn plays a central role in Adam's motivation. It would be notable to discuss how each of these relationships contribute to Adam's mental health.

The Memory of Light by Francisco **X.** Stork (2017)

Summary

Sixteen-year-old Vicky Cruz awakens in the hospital after attempting suicide. While in the Group Therapy Healing (GTH) she meets with the therapist, Dr. Desai; Mona, her roommate in the mental ward who has bipolar disorder; Emilio (EM) with anger-management issues and possibly intermittent explosive disorder; and the thoughtful, spiritual Gabriel, who exhibits schizophrenia. As the group grows closer, they provide support and acceptance for each other as they help Vicky become strong enough to face her father, help her Nana, and find her place in her world.

Mental health issues: Depression, suicidal ideation, bipolar disorder, anger issues, schizophrenia.

Why the Novel Was Chosen

This novel features a female protagonist as well as another female and two male lead characters, all of whom are multidimensional—not simply defined by their illness. Readers learn about the lives of the characters outside the hospital setting. This novel also includes intergenerational characters and multicultural, mainly Latinx, characters. The male author is Latino and lives with depression. The incorporation of multiple main characters may appeal to readers. This novel portrays a positive exploration of mental health services and ends with plans for treatment or recovery for the four main characters.

Look-Fors Based on Reading Literacy Lessons

The novel is narrated in the first person. Since there are four main characters, the book club discussion can focus on the advantages of one character narrating the story and of providing that character's perspective as opposed to having the story told in third person or even from multiple perspectives. Readers first meet Vicky through her suicide note to Juanita, and they might discuss why the author introduces her this way and what they learn about her character from her letter and then her time in the hospital. Readers can also discuss what they learn about Vicky through her interactions with other characters and how her goals change throughout the novel as she becomes centered and more attached to her therapy group members.

The relationships among the characters are significant in this novel, especially Vicky's relationship with each of them, not only the group members and her therapist but also her Nana, father, sister, and her former best friend. Some of those relationships change during the time period of the novel. Vicky's relationship with her mother, and comparison with the relationships of her father and sister with her mother, during Vicky's mental illness can provide topics of conversation.

Look-Fors Based on Mental Health Literacy Lessons

Each character's difficulties are revealed through their interaction with Vicky. Likewise, each character provides their version of Vicky's symptoms, giving the reader a variety of perspectives to discuss. Specifically, readers can discuss how Vicky comes to understand depression after being "diagnosed" by Mona. Vicky's awareness of her symptoms and description of the "yellow fog" provide insight into the process of coming to grips with a diagnosis of depression.

Vicky's goals change throughout the novel as she comes to understand depression. Initially, she has no hope for receiving help and seeing improvement, but she comes to see the possibility of remission and recovery. Through Vicky's father, the reader can see common stereotypes about mental illness and inpatient treatment.

Relationships are the central focus of Vicky's awareness of and initial recovery from depression. Readers can discuss the impact of depression on Vicky's withdrawal from her friends and family. Readers can also note how the grief from her mother's death and the complicated relationship with her older sister serve to highlight how various relationship stressors impact the development of Vicky's mental health concerns.

Readers can note that Vicky's home environment provides material support but not emotional support. Considering Vicky's thoughts about her resources in comparison to those of Mona, EM, and Gabriel can lead students to a discussion about the various stressors in each character's background. The environment at the hospital, and at the ranch, can also be discussed in relation to such supportive factors as the safety of the group, the sense of contributing to others, and the structure of each day.

AFTER-READING RESEARCH AND PRESENTATIONS

One advantage of book club reading is that, while reading only one novel, students can hear about five different novels and the mental health issues depicted in each through post-reading presentations; therefore, each book club can conclude their book study by collaborating and creating a 20-minute presentation of their novel and its mental health focus.

Preparing for and presenting an after-reading presentation allows readers to discover what they know and synthesize, expand that understanding, and then share that knowledge with others. Presentations not only relate information learned but also guide readers to rethink the meaning of this learning and connect it to other learning and their developing views of the world in which they live.

After the final reading and text discussion meeting, teachers can collaborate with the school's media specialist and mental health professional to facilitate each book club's research of the mental health foci addressed in their novel, including symptoms, recommended prevention and self-help strategies, current statistics, and available help for adolescents experiencing these issues. Students can also connect their research to the young adult title read, presenting an overview of their novels to the class.

Some project suggestions would be to present a documentary, infomercial, talk show, skit, or I Am poetry. Students can also be encouraged to create their own ideas for presentations. In each presentation, book club members can include facts from their research and a synopsis of their novel, including setting, characters, and plot elements, especially the central conflict(s).

For example, a talk show may feature a host or facilitator to introduce the guests: the main characters of the novel and a mental health expert. The expert can share information about the mental health issues addressed in the novel, including statistics and facts, while the characters could answer questions posed about how challenges were handled and their relationships with other characters. Or, in a presentation based on I Am poetry, characters can present their individual I Am poem and a student acting as a mental health professional might present their I Am poem as a representative of the profession or one that incorporated the research reviewed.

CONCLUSION

Reading novels involving mental health topics through book clubs opens the opportunity to share and discuss personal interpretations and experiences on this sometimes-sensitive topic. Book clubs offer countless advantages to individual students. Book clubs are social and supportive; small groups lead to deeper, collaborative, and more meaningful discussions, particularly on sensitive topics. Having a choice of novels and the requirement to read the text as a precursor to participation, book clubs can lead to increased motivation to read. In addition, students can read multiple formats of texts at the same time: prose, verse novels, and graphic novels across multiple mental health topics. Moreover, through the after-reading presentations, readers have the opportunity to learn about five or six other novels. Most important, the collaborative skills exercised in book club reading and meeting can prepare students for authentic interactions.

REFERENCES

Anderson, L. H. (2009). *Wintergirls*. New York: Viking Books for Young Readers.
Centers for Disease Control. (2020, June 15). *Data and statistics on children's mental health*. https://www.cdc.gov/childrensmentalhealth/data.html

Corinne Duyvis [@corinneduyvis]. (n.d.). *Tweets* [Twitter profile]. Twitter. Retrieved April 23, 2021, from https://twitter.com/corinneduyvis?ref_src =twsrc%5Egoogle%7Ctwcamp%5Eserp%7Ctwgr%5Eauthor

Furnham, A., & Swami, V. (2018). Mental health literacy: A review of what it is and why it matters. *International Perspectives in Psychology*, 7(4), 240–57. https://doi.org/10.1037/ipp0000094

Holman, L. F., MacGillivray, L., Salem, W., & Tarbett, L. B. (2019). Book club groups to aid relational connection and trust among addicted trauma survivors. *Journal of Creativity in Mental Health*, 14(1), 37–53. https://doi.org/10 .1080/15401383.2018.1502706

National Eating Disorders Association. (2020, May 8). *Statistics and research on eating disorders.* https://www.nationaleatingdisorders.org/statistics-research -eating-disorders

National Institute of Mental Health. (2017, November). *Eating disorders.* https:// www.nimh.nih.gov/health/statistics/eating-disorders.shtml#part_155062

Rainfield, C. (2010). *Scars.* Lodi, NJ: WestSide Books.

Roessing, L. (2007). Losing the fear of sharing control. *Middle School Journal*, 38(3), 44–51. https://doi.org/10.1080/00940771.2007.11461583

Roessing, L. (2009). *The write to read: Response journals that increase comprehension.* Thousand Oaks, CA: Corwin.

Roessing, L. (2019). *Talking texts: A teachers' guide to book clubs across the curriculum.* Lanham, MD: Rowman & Littlefield.

Sevinc, G. (2019). Healing mental health through reading: Bibliotherapy. *Current Approaches in Psychiatry*, 11(4), 483–95. https://doi.org/10.18863/ pgy.474083

Sones, S. (2016). *Saving Red.* New York: HarperTeen.

Stork, F. (2017). *The memory of light.* New York: Arthur A. Levine Books.

Stork, F. (2018). Captain, my captain. In M. Nijkamp (Ed.), *Unbroken: Stories starring disabled teens* (pp. 157–76). New York: Farrar, Straus & Giroux.

Toten, T. (2013). *The unlikely hero of room 13B.* Toronto: Doubleday Canada.

Wilder, P. (2019). "Conversations with myself": Literacy as a conscious tool of healing. *English Journal*, 108(3), 60–66.

ADDITIONAL RESOURCES ON MENTAL HEALTH

American Academy of Child and Adolescent Psychiatry (AACAP): https://www
.aacap.org/
American Foundation for Suicide Prevention (AFSP): https://afsp.org/
American Psychological Association (APA): https://www.apa.org/
Anxiety and Depression Association of America (ADAA): https://adaa.org/
Association for Size Diversity and Health (ASDAH): https://asdah.org/health
-at-every-size-haes-approach/
Centers for Disease Control and Prevention (CDC): https://www.cdc.gov/men
talhealth/index.htm
International OCD Foundation: https://iocdf.org/about-ocd/
National Alliance on Mental Illness (NAMI): https://www.nami.org/
National Association of School Psychologists (NASP): https://www.nasponline
.org/
National Child Traumatic Stress Network (NCTSN): https://www.nctsn.org/
National Eating Disorders Association (NEDA): https://www.nationaleating
disorders.org/
National Institute of Mental Health (NIMH): https://www.nimh.nih.gov/
Substance Use and Mental Health Services Administration (SAMHSA): https://
www.samhsa.gov/

INDEX

ABOUT THE EDITORS
AND CONTRIBUTORS

ABOUT THE EDITORS

Brooke Eisenbach is associate professor of middle and secondary education at Lesley University. She has coedited several books, including *Queer Adolescent Literature as a Complement to the English Language Arts Curriculum* and *The Online Classroom: Resources for Effective Middle Level Virtual Education*. Her research on middle-level education, virtual education, and young adult literature has been published in such books and top-tier journals as *Voices from the Middle*, *Research in Middle Level Education Online*, *The Clearing House*, and *English Journal*. Eisenbach is a former middle-level English and YA Literature teacher and virtual school teacher with more than 10 years of experience. She has received several teaching awards, notably the National Council of Teachers of English (NCTE) Outstanding Middle Level Educator Award.

Jason Scott Frydman is assistant professor of psychology at Lesley University. He is a nationally certified school psychologist and registered drama therapist, and has extensive clinical experience working with middle-level and high school students for the past 13 years. His research focuses on trauma-informed programming for K–12 students and the implementation and use of the creative arts therapies in the school setting. His scholarship has been published across a variety of peer-reviewed journals, including *Children & Schools*, *Psychology in the Schools*, *Arts in Psychotherapy*, and *Drama Therapy Review* (*DTR*). Frydman serves on the editorial boards of *School Psychology Review*; *Translational Issues in Psychological Science*; and *DTR*, for which he guest coedited the schools-focused special issue (2019). He has been recognized for his outstanding professional contributions by the American Academy of School Psychology and the North American Drama Therapy Association.

ABOUT THE CONTRIBUTORS

Arianna Banack is a doctoral candidate at the University of Tennessee, Knoxville (UTK), in the literacy studies program with a specialization in children's and young adult literature. She is currently serving as one of the assistant editors of the *ALAN Review*. Her research interests focus on the connections between adolescent reading engagement and young adult literature. She has had articles published in several peer-reviewed journals, including *English Journal* and the *ALAN Review*. Prior to enrolling at UTK, Banack taught high school English for a large district in Connecticut.

Terry Benton is assistant professor of English at Youngstown State University. She earned a BS in education from Youngstown State University with majors in elementary education and secondary education–English, an MA in English from Youngstown State University, and a PhD in curriculum and instruction from Kent State University. Benton's professional interests include children's and young adult literature, diversity in youth literature, access to literature, literacy instruction, and the teaching of writing.

Daniela Bustamante is a licensed creative arts therapist and psychiatric registered nurse based in Los Angeles, California. She has worked in various mental health treatment settings and specializes in working with adolescents. Daniela has also presented on the role of cultural and intersectional identities in mental health treatment for organizations including the North American Drama Therapy Association, New York University, and Molloy College. Bustamante is currently pursuing her master's degree in family psychiatric mental health nursing at California State University, Los Angeles.

Caitlin Corrieri is an English teacher at the Chenery Middle School in Belmont, Massachusetts, where she has taught grades 6, 7, and 8 for the past 12 years. She received her bachelor's degree from Boston College and her master's degree from Providence College, and she is working toward licensure as a literacy specialist. She is an elected executive board member for the New England Association of Teachers of English (NEATE), where she also promotes their events on social media. Corrieri has presented on the subject of social emotional learning through young adult literature at professional conferences including the New England League of Middle Schools (NELMS), the Association for Middle Level Education (AMLE), and the National Council of Teachers of English (NCTE).

MaryBeth DeGennaro is a seasoned educator with 18 years in public schools as an elementary teacher and a high school librarian. She is also certified as a public librarian. Prior to becoming a teacher, she worked in publishing in a variety of capacities for Baker & Taylor, Amazon.com, and Random House.

Grace Enriquez is professor of language and literacy at Lesley University in Cambridge, Massachusetts. A former English language arts teacher, reading specialist, and literacy staff developer, she has focused scholarship on children's literature for social justice; reader response; critical literacies; intersections of literacies, identities, and embodiment; and the teaching of writing. Grace is the children's literature editor for the *Reading Teacher*, coauthor of the School Library Journal blog *The Classroom Bookshelf*, and coauthor/editor of several books. Her work has appeared in various national and international peer-reviewed journals. Enriquez also serves on national literacy committees and editorial review boards, and she has received grants from the American Library Association, the Children's Literature Assembly, and the National Council of Teachers of English. Her current work explores how culturally responsive and sustaining pedagogy can support students' multimodal reader responses.

Elyana Genovese has been a school counselor at a middle school in Northern Virginia for four years. She received her bachelor's degree from James Madison University and her master's degree in school counseling from George Washington University. She has contributed to a published group activities book for the Association for Specialists in Group Work (ASGW). Her favorite part of her job is connecting with students and seeing their academic and social/emotional achievements. Genovese loves soccer and coaches the girls' varsity soccer team at a nearby high school.

Mary Mae Kelly is a clinical social worker in Michigan's Saginaw Bay area. She completed her bachelor of social work degree at Saginaw Valley State University in 2008 and earned a master of social work degree from Michigan State University in 2009. Kelly started her career in mental health with inpatient treatment settings and transitioned fully to outpatient settings in 2013. She has been comprehensively trained in dialectical behavior therapy. Other areas of specialty include trauma, grief and loss, and mood and anxiety disorders. She and her partner love spending time in the outdoors and with their two dogs and one cat.

Elsie Lindy Olan is associate professor and track coordinator for secondary English language arts in the School of Teacher Education at the University of Central Florida. Her work has been published in *English Education, English Leadership Quarterly, Research in the Teaching of English, Education and Learning Research Journal, Argentinian Journal of Applied Linguistics*, and *Language Arts*. Her current research on teacher education, leadership, and diversity is shared in a coedited book series, Transformative Pedagogies for Teacher Education. Olan has presented her work and research at conferences in Mexico, Spain, the United Kingdom, Japan, and the United States.

Michelle Pate is assistant professor of art therapy at Lesley University. Pate holds an MA in community counseling from Wayne State

University and a doctorate of art therapy from Mount Mary University. Before becoming an educator, Michelle worked in community mental health with families and children in Detroit, Michigan. Her research and pedagogy focus on undergraduate art therapy education, inclusion, and advocacy.

Kia Jane Richmond is professor of English at Northern Michigan University in Marquette, Michigan, and directs the English education program and supervises student teachers in Michigan and Wisconsin. Her research focuses on teacher-student relationships, psychology and young adult literature, and English education pedagogy. Her publications have appeared in *English Education, Journal of Literacy and Language Education*, the *ALAN Review, Language Arts Journal of Michigan*, and *Composition Studies*. Richmond's latest book, *Mental Illness in Young Adult Literature: Exploring Real Struggles through Fictional Characters*, was published in 2019.

Allen Rigell is a board-certified psychiatrist practicing in Knoxville, Tennessee. Dr. Rigell has extensive experience treating anxiety, depression, attention deficit disorders, bipolar disorder, sleep problems, trauma-related stress disorders, and other mental health disorders. He received his BA from Emory University and his MD from East Tennessee State University. He completed his residency in psychiatry at the University of Wisconsin in Madison. In addition to his professional interests, Dr. Rigell also has a personal interest in athletics and in stories like Mickey Catalan's. He was captain of his baseball team in college and played in the college World Series.

Amanda Rigell is a doctoral student and graduate teaching associate in literacy education at the University of Tennessee, Knoxville. Her research interests include instructional decision making, reading motivation, the reading-writing connection, and models of teacher resistance. Rigell has been published in several peer-reviewed journals, including *English Journal* and *American Educational Research Journal*. She is a licensed reading specialist and has 13 years of experience as a middle and high school classroom teacher.

Lesley Roessing was a middle and high school teacher for 20 years and the founding director of the Coastal Savannah Writing Project at Armstrong State University where she was also a senior lecturer in the College of Education. She also served as a literacy consultant for a K–8 school and has presented workshops for professional organizations and provided professional development for many school districts. Lesley served as past editor of *Connections*, the award-winning GCTE journal. As a columnist for *AMLE Magazine* of the Association for Middle Level Education, she authored the "Writing to Learn" columns. Roessing has written articles on literacy for a variety of educational journals. She is the author of five books for educators—*The Write to Read, Bridging the Gap, No More "Us" and "Them," Comma Quest*, and *Talking Texts*—and has contributed to four books on writing and literature.

Katie Sciurba is assistant professor of literacy education at San Diego State University (SDSU) and director of the SDSU Literacy Center. Her research focuses on the intersections of young people's identities and literacy practices, popular culture as a vehicle for literacy instruction, and representations of race, gender, and current/recent historical events in children's literature. Sciurba holds a PhD in English education from New York University. Her scholarly work has been published in such venues as *Teachers College Record, Journal of Literacy Research, Journal of Adolescent & Adult Literacy*, and *Children's Literature in Education*; she is the author of texts for children, including the picture-book, *Oye, Celia! A Song for Celia Cruz* (2007).

Jeff Spanke is assistant professor of English at Ball State University where he teaches courses in young adult literature, rhetoric and composition, and English teaching methods. He is a former high school English teacher who served rural students in northwest and central Indiana. Spanke's current scholarship examines the roles of citizenship and civic identity in secondary English language arts instruction, as well as the social constructions of teachers and students, particularly in "rurban" spaces. His past writings have focused on teenage religiosity, professional development, and the role of reflection in teacher education.

Jessica Traylor has worked as a school psychologist since 2003. She is the coauthor of *Real Girls: Shifting Perceptions on Identity, Relationships, and the Media*, a group counseling guide. Dr. Traylor has presented at national and international conferences covering such topics as collaboration, service-learning, rural education, self-regulated learning, self-efficacy, experiential learning, mentoring, trauma and resilience, and youth mental health. Dr. Traylor has been a professor since 2014. She is currently an assistant professor of psychology and the coordinator of service-learning at Gordon State College. She also serves as a lead affiliate faculty for Ohio Christian University. Her research interests include adverse childhood experiences, resilience, service-learning, and civic engagement. She enjoys teaching courses in psychology of adjustment, human growth and development, and trauma and resilience. In addition to her formal degrees, Dr. Traylor is also a certified yoga instructor, holistic nutrition coach, therapeutic drumming instructor, and Hellenistic astrologer.

Sara Tyner received her graduate degree from Appalachian State University in Boone, North Carolina, and has practiced as a mental health clinician for nine years. In addition to her time working with folks in Appalachia, Tyner has practiced primarily in rural settings in both North Carolina and Indiana, focusing on the uninsured and underinsured population. Sara currently practices at a small nonprofit in Lafayette, Indiana, working with those who have financial barriers and obstacles.

Laura L. Wood is a registered drama therapist, board-certified trainer, licensed clinical mental health counselor, licensed creative arts therapist, and a certified child life specialist. Dr. Wood is associate professor at Lesley University. Prior to being a full-time professor, Dr. Wood was the lead therapist at an eating disorder and trauma treatment center where she facilitated individual, group, and family therapy. Her focus and research areas include the treatment of trauma and dissociation, eating disorders, attachment, recovery, grief/loss, and the use of therapeutic theater. Dr. Wood presents, publishes, supervises, and consults nationally and internationally. She sees clients in private practice and facilitates intensive healing retreats for people in recovery.

Sherri Harper Woods is assistant professor of social work and the Master of Social Work Program coordinator at Youngstown State University. She completed undergraduate studies at Youngstown State University, the Master of Social Science Administration at Case Western Reserve University, and the Doctor of Ministry in Formational Counseling at Ashland Theological Seminary. Woods's professional interests include curriculum development, trauma recovery, integrating spirituality into the treatment process, service-learning and civic engagement, mind and body interventions, and continuing education development.

Made in the USA
Coppell, TX
05 May 2022

77421584R00132